EFFORTLESS

G000129432

DR CAROLINE SHREEVE qualified after training at St Mary's Hospital, London, and at the Royal College of Surgeons in Dublin. She has been principal partner in general practice in London, a locum and out-of-hours deputy throughout the UK, and has worked overseas, mostly in South Africa and Australia. Nutritional and physical fitness, psychological therapies and complementary medicine are her chief medical interests. Caroline has written extensively for newspapers and magazines and also has a long list of books on health to her credit, the most recent of which, *Fat-burner Foods* (2002), was serialized in the London *Evening Standard*.

Caroline lives in Pembrokeshire with her pug and two cats.

Overcoming Common Problems Series

A full list of titles is available from Sheldon Press,
1 Marylebone Road, London NW1 4DU, and on our website at
www.sheldonpress.co.uk

Overcoming Common Problems Series

Overcoming Common Problems Series

How to Untangle Your Emotional Knots
Dr Windy Dryden and Jack Gordon

Hysterectomy
Suzie Hayman

Is HRT Right for You?
Dr Anne MacGregor

Jealousy
Dr Paul Hauck

Lifting Depression the Balanced Way
Dr Lindsay Corrie

Living with Asthma
Dr Robert Youngson

Living with Crohn's Disease
Dr Joan Gomez

Living with Diabetes
Dr Joan Gomez

Living with Fibromyalgia
Christine Craggs-Hinton

Living with Grief
Dr Tony Lake

Living with Heart Disease
Victor Marks, Dr Monica Lewis and Dr Gerald Lewis

Living with High Blood Pressure
Dr Tom Smith

Living with Hughes Syndrome
Triona Holden

Living with Nut Allergies
Karen Evennett

Living with Osteoarthritis
Dr Patricia Gilbert

Living with Osteoporosis
Dr Joan Gomez

Living with a Stoma
Dr Craig White

Make Up or Break Up: Making the Most of Your Marriage
Mary Williams

Making Friends with Your Stepchildren
Rosemary Wells

Motor Neurone Disease – A Family Affair
Dr David Oliver

Overcoming Anger
Dr Windy Dryden

Overcoming Anxiety
Dr Windy Dryden

Overcoming Back Pain
Dr Tom Smith

Overcoming Depression
Dr Windy Dryden and Sarah Opie

Overcoming Guilt
Dr Windy Dryden

Overcoming Jealousy
Dr Windy Dryden

Overcoming Procrastination
Dr Windy Dryden

Overcoming Shame
Dr Windy Dryden

Overcoming Your Addictions
Dr Windy Dryden and
Dr Walter Matweychuk

The Parkinson's Disease Handbook
Dr Richard Godwin-Austen

The PMS Diet Book
Karen Evennett

A Positive Thought for Every Day
Dr Windy Dryden

Rheumatoid Arthritis
Mary-Claire Mason and Dr Elaine Smith

Shift Your Thinking, Change Your Life
Mo Shapiro

Stress and Depression in Children and Teenagers
Vicky Maud

Stress at Work
Mary Hartley

The Stress Workbook
Joanna Gutmann

Successful Au Pairs
Hilli Matthews

Ten Steps to Positive Living
Dr Windy Dryden

Think Your Way to Happiness
Dr Windy Dryden and Jack Gordon

The Traveller's Good Health Guide
Ted Lankester

Understanding Obsessions and Compulsions
Dr Frank Tallis

Understanding Sex and Relationships
Rosemary Stones

Understanding Your Personality
Patricia Hedges

Work–Life Balance
Gordon and Ronni Lamont

Your Man's Health
Fiona Marshall

Overcoming Common Problems

Effortless Exercise

Dr Caroline Shreeve

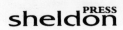

First published in Great Britain in 2003 by
Sheldon Press
1 Marylebone Road
London NW1 4DU

Copyright © Caroline Shreeve 2003

All rights reserved. No part of this book may be reproduced
or transmitted in any form or by any means, electronic or
mechanical, including photocopying, recording, or by any
information storage and retrieval system, without permission
in writing from the publisher.

British Library Cataloguing-in-Publication Data

A catalogue record for this book is available from the British Library

ISBN 0–85969–872–6

1 3 5 7 9 10 8 6 4 2

Typeset by Deltatype Limited, Birkenhead, Merseyside
Printed in Great Britain by Biddles Ltd
www.biddles.co.uk

Contents

Introduction

Do you enjoy exercising? Almost certainly not or you would not be reading this book. In fact if, like me, you're a couch potato at heart, you probably detest the idea of anything requiring you to be vertically mobile – particularly on a regular basis! Life, you may feel, is far too demanding for you to waste precious leisure hours you normally spend reading, chatting or watching TV working up a sweat.

You may secretly admire your more energetic friends, though, and feel that you too would benefit from a trimmer figure, more supple muscles and joints, and that glowing complexion that seems to come from more fresh air and oxygen. It's just that you haven't exercised for years, constantly feel exhausted and really haven't the time to include exercise in your life.

Well, you can forget about sweat for a start! According to an old saying, horses sweat, men perspire and ladies merely glow. Better still, it is possible to build more activity into your life without doing any of these – unless, of course, you choose to. You can achieve this happy state without setting aside lots of large blocks of time a week from your already brimming schedule.

The secret truly is softee, softee, catchee monkey – creep up on yourself with a few minutes here and there, prolonging things you already do or introducing something new that you really enjoy. Before you know it, you will be reducing the risks of a slothful lifestyle and gaining many positive health benefits too.

Risks

Is the couch potato's lifestyle really to blame for all the health hazards with which it is often linked? Are we instead just urged to take more exercise by a sadistic 'health police' who would, given the chance, dictate what we eat, when and how we exercise – and perhaps even when and with whom we sleep?

The fact is that lying and sitting about all day, delightful though these are, can seriously damage your health. Data on the health trends of societies in the developed world, and research studies into the commonest causes of death and their links to diet and lifestyle, have established this fact beyond any doubt.

Some of the risks of being inactive are due to surplus bodyweight; other, more general ones, result from misuse and underuse of the body as a whole.

The hazards of being overweight

We're talking here not about plumpness or being slightly overweight, but about obesity. To qualify as obese you need to be 20 per cent or more above the upper limit of the desirable weight range for your sex, build and height (this is further explained in Chapter 2, pages 24–27). Briefly, the possible health implications of obesity are as follows.

Life-threatening diseases strongly linked to obesity

These include high blood pressure and its complications, such as angina, heart attacks, heart failure and stroke, deep vein thrombosis (DVT), kidney disorders, Types I and II diabetes, and ovarian, breast and bowel cancer. Recent figures show us that obesity has tripled over the past two decades and that half of all adults in the UK are now overweight, one in five being obese. Obesity doubles a person's chances of dying from heart disease. Obese women are 27 times more at risk from developing diabetes and have 50 per cent increased chance of suffering from breast cancer. Obese men are a third more likely to die from cancer.

Alice, 58
'I gained weight after having each of my 3 children, and again at the menopause when I was 52. I stopped work and was far less active – more pounds crept on over the next three years. Finally I weighed 14 stone (89 kg) which, at only 5 foot 4 inches (about 1.53 m) high, meant I was seriously overweight (i.e. obese). I stopped going to my GP for annual checkups because I knew she'd want me to diet, and I just hadn't the willpower. But then I started to notice chest pains when I hurried for a bus, carried heavy shopping or got angry or overexcited. My husband insisted I see our doctor – in fact he came with me and made sure I told her all my symptoms.

'My blood pressure was high at 170 over 105 and an ECG [electrocardiograph heart tracing] indicated that my heart was under strain. My blood cholesterol level was also raised. Doctor P diagnosed angina and said I simply had to become more active – sitting about all day was helping to fur up the coronary arteries that supply the heart muscle and the angina was a warning signal of a pending heart attack. She prescribed blood pressure tablets and asked me to start a gentle daily walking programme. I also watched what I ate and cut down my consumption of saturated fats.

'I now walk for about half an hour four or five times a week. I reached my goal weight of 9½ stone (60 kg) last Christmas and no longer need blood pressure medication. My blood cholesterol has normalized too. Angina is just a bad memory – I feel so well, and have so much more energy.'

Other disorders

Though not life-threatening, certain other disorders are caused or worsened by obesity, including gall bladder disease, osteoarthritis, asthma, skin infections and other rashes, chronic backache, sciatica, hernias, haemorrhoids, varicose veins, heartburn and other digestive problems, period problems and failure to conceive.

Ann, 40

'My husband and I had been trying to start a family for three years when we finally went to our doctor for help. We had put this off for some time – I was 36 – and afraid that my age was the reason for my failure to get pregnant; whereas Clive (aged 35) feared he might be to blame – he had had one of his testicles removed following a football injury at the age of 22 and blamed what he suspected was his low sperm count.

'But we were amazed when the specialist we were referred to told us that my being overweight could be the underlying problem. I had always been heavy – standing 5 foot 7 inches (1.54 m) I had weighed 16 stone (101 kg) since before we married – and had never thought much about it. I suppose I was so used to being tired all the time, puffing up stairs and up slopes and sweating heavily in warm surroundings, that I had just got used to it. The gynaecologist explained that thick layers of surplus body fat can adversely affect a woman's hormonal cycle and her chances of becoming pregnant.

'He gave me simple instructions for becoming more active – we were already eating quite healthily – and I saw our GP once a month so he could monitor my weight loss. Clive and I went walking for half an hour four times a week and swimming at the weekend as well. Once I gave up being a couch potato, I started to enjoy my new lifestyle and the pounds dropped away, month after month.

'I had been at my goal weight of 9½ stone (60 kg) for only three months when a pregnancy test proved positive and our baby daughter was born healthily nine months later. We couldn't get over this simple solution, when we had imagined we'd be spending thousands of pounds on IVF to cure infertility.'

The psychological effects of obesity, which can be equally damaging, range from poor self-esteem, social phobias and low libido to lack of confidence and even agoraphobia. Obesity can also exact a dreadful toll on one's love life. Feeling self-consciously fat dampens our desire and can adversely affect relationships – for instance, when one or other partner becomes reluctant to undress or make love with the light on. Conversely, few of us would deny the reduced allure of a fat-laden partner or lover. Being horrendously fat also interferes with the basic mechanics of lovemaking.

Joanna, 25
'I had never had agoraphobia before – in fact, I did not even know what it was. I was a life and soul of the party girl – into everything and forever socializing – but then I had always been a perfect size 10. I did not know what had hit me when the pounds piled on when I was expecting the twins, and after they were delivered I found I had gained 4 stone (25 kg) and was a size 16.

'I had an attack of postnatal depression a month afterwards – it slowly got better with antidepressants, but my weight had gone up further and I became reluctant to go out. Pete, my husband, tried to get a babysitter and make me come out once a week at least for the evening, but I had been in for weeks looking after the babies by that time and lost the confidence.

'I just couldn't bear the thought of people in the supermarket, the pub, friends and family seeing me look like Mrs Blobby . . . It got so bad that I needed psychotherapy and further antidepressants and contact with a local agoraphobia support group, which helped me gradually to take a few steps outside and, much later, to go shopping if accompanied.

'Ultimately, I lost the weight by following a strict diet plan I found on the Internet. But being fat altered my personality for a time and next time I get pregnant, I am definitely going to see that I do not pile on the pounds as I did first time round.'

Other health risks linked to chronic, long-term inactivity

These include degenerating bones, joints and muscles, osteoporosis (for both sexes, but especially women), poor self-image, premature ageing, poor stamina and immunity, anxiety-related disorders and clinical depression.

Joanne, 20

'I was always very keen on sports, especially tennis and hockey, while I was at school, but an accident on the playing field meant I had to give these up for over a year while my knee injury was investigated and treated. I was actually advised to remain fairly active and given an exercise schedule that would keep me physically fit and strengthen my knee ligaments, but I did not follow it. I was so upset at having to give up competitive sports that I went into a decline – sat about all day watching the television and reading magazines. It was my gap year anyway, so I could just give in to my misery as much as I liked.

'I didn't put on weight – I come from a really skinny family and must have a high metabolic rate – but my mood got lower and lower, and each day I was spending longer and longer in bed. There just did not appear to be anything worth getting up for . . .

'Finally, my mother asked our GP to visit and, after chatting with me, he diagnosed clinical depression. My parents and I were amazed – none of us had ever suffered with anything like that before. I was given a course of a low-dose antidepressant and advised by a physiotherapist on gentle exercise techniques to help me regain my fitness before starting Uni the following October. I didn't realize the exercise part of the treatment was so important – my mood and energy levels zoomed upwards for months after I came off the tablets and I began to see the point of life again. Like so many people (and at least two of my friends), an accident had triggered a spell of inactivity, which in turn had spiralled into depression. Exercise was the key to my recovery.'

1
Aerobic Exercise

The type of activity most of us think of in connection with the word 'exercise', is aerobic. This variety offers the most health benefits and best combats the risks of a couch potato's lifestyle. However, if the very word conjures up visions of smug, Lycra-clad skinnies doing intricate step routines to blaring pop music, then you share my – and many other people's – vision of hell. Such images deter thousands of us from getting up and literally saving our lives. All 'aerobic' means is utilizing oxygen from the air, so *any* activity can qualify as aerobic, provided it increases the amount of oxygen we inhale while doing it. It is quite unnecessary to jog down the road in full sight of the neighbours or walk up 20 flights of stairs at work if the lift is in perfect working order.

We'll be seeing later in this chapter that what is aerobic for us varies from one individual to another. We should never exercise so vigorously that we can't talk while doing it! There's a safe, dependable formula for working out our own aerobic requirement, based on age, pulse rate and health. Meanwhile, the chief gains are physical and emotional – you *can* look forward to doing something every day that puts up your pulse rate and makes you breathe more quickly.

Physical benefits

Weight control
Probably the best recognized (and sought-after) benefit is that normal bodyweight can be achieved, which is necessary for a healthy heart, lungs and circulation. However fat and unfit we are, becoming even slightly more active in small ways significantly reduces our risks of heart attack or stroke. Fighting the flab also lessens our chances of developing all the other fat-related complaints we've already looked at and helps prevent damage to weight-bearing joints, such as lower spine, hips, knees and ankles.

Increased stamina
This is one of the first benefits to appear after starting to become more active. We soon notice that we become less breathless when

1

climbing stairs, vacuuming, hurrying for a bus or train, carrying a baby or toddler and/or lugging heavy shopping. Demanding physical chores – digging, mowing the lawn, cleaning the car – also become less exhausting. Simple, unalarming, enjoyable pastimes soon get us breathing more deeply. Using more of the available lung power in this way increases the amount of oxygen-rich air at our disposal (oxygen is the flame that lights the fire that burns body fat – among other things) and gets rid of more carbon dioxide, water and other waste. A few extra minutes of activity included in our day – here and there – also strengthens the heart, helping it work at maximum efficiency, which in turn improves the delivery of fresh blood to all the tissues of the body.

Increased strength

This means that bones, ligaments and tendons toughen up and our muscles work more efficiently. Our thigh muscles, calves and feet, buttocks and spine tire less easily if we do small, regular amounts of weight-bearing activities, such as brisk walking, dancing or skating. The muscle groups of the upper part of the body – spine, chest, shoulders, upper back, upper and lower arms – are also strengthened by skipping, swimming, rowing, horse riding, dancing and racquet games.

Increased lean muscle mass

When muscles strengthen, they increase in size, which in turn increases the amount of lean body tissue at the expense of surplus fat. This means that we end up leaner, meaner and trimmer and burn fat more readily. Muscular tissue, weighing more than fat, can apparently slow down weight loss in the fight against obesity. We look slimmer, though, even when the scales remain at a certain weight for a few weeks. Having more lean muscle tissue turns us into a fat-burning machine as the metabolism speeds up, burning stored fat and food fuel more efficiently.

Increased energy levels

Besides improved stamina and use of food fuel, our energy levels receive a boost as a result of better digestion and waste elimination. Also, the delivery of oxygen and nutrients to the heart and body muscles, brain, nerves and vital organs is enhanced due to the improvements in the circulation that occur.

Sleep

The quality of sleep improves when we build more physical demands into our day. Becoming physically tired from regular workouts cuts the risks of tossing and turning throughout the night due to worry or sleep disturbances (such as early morning waking) that can accompany depression.

Anti-ageing

If we lose surplus body fat, strengthen and refine our muscles and improve our overall fitness (while boosting our self-esteem and feelings of vitality), we both look and feel more attractive. There is some evidence that regular aerobic exercise also stimulates the production and release of growth hormone from the pituitary gland in the brain, in older as well as younger people. Supplements of human growth hormone (HGH) have been used to promote youthfulness, maintain a trim and lean body, boost vitality and improve the healthy (and youthful) functioning of the brain.

Improved circulation and oxygen and nutrient delivery to the main body organs and skin also improves our appearance. The skin clears and complexion improves, the tongue loses its white coating and shows a healthy strawberry pink. Improved nourishment shows in the condition of skin, hair and nails. The kidneys, liver and lymphatic system are on top form, ensuring that we excrete waste material and toxic substances promptly. Moreover, the reproductive system works well and, with increased self-esteem and improved body image, plus more energy, sex can only improve.

Women who stay physically active suffer less from premenstrual syndrome (PMS), period pains, disorders of pregnancy and menopausal symptoms. Men stay alert and active – and often sexually potent – into advanced old age. Both sexes, when fit, flexible and free from anxiety and depression, are more inclined to share and enjoy lovemaking well into their later years. Satisfaction of this sort tends to be reflected externally, although it is more than skin deep. Men's and women's skin and complexions benefit from all these aspects of renewed health, showing more of a glow and fewer lines and wrinkles.

Mind and emotions

Mental alertness

Exercise boosts brain power! Recent research has shown a link between becoming more physically active and our ability to reason

3

and think. An improved supply of blood, oxygen and nutrients to the brain, a greater sense of well-being, coping better with stress and tension, greater freedom from anxiety and depression and better-quality sleep are all thought to contribute to this. The functions of the brain that improve as a result of regular activity include short-term memory (the type mainly affected by brain ageing disorders such as dementia and Alzheimer's disease), our planning abilities, organizational skills and the ability to do several different things at once.

These benefits were discovered during a research study comparing the effects of exercise and antidepressant drugs on depression. Attention, concentration and the performance of manual skills requiring mental input, however, were unaffected. The study, named SMILE (Standard Medical Intervention and Long-term Exercise), reported in the *Journal of Ageing and Physical Activity*, involved 156 people aged between 50 and 77 with a major depressive disorder. The patients with milder depression showed the most improvement, both moodwise and in terms of their mental functioning.

Improved stress tolerance
Feeling livelier and more balanced emotionally due to regular aerobic activity leads to a more stable mood and improved capacity to cope with stressful situations. Success in any life-enhancing skill normally makes us feel good; but becoming more active also provides an outlet for the knot of tension and frustration we can all experience. A brief walk in the open air, ten minutes' swimming, releases the mental and physical tension triggered by release of the stress hormones adrenaline and noradrenaline.

Feeling on top of the world
All the benefits so far described combine to boost that feeling of *wellness*, vitality, that we can cope with all things and an enthusiasm for life that we all experience when we improve our overall fitness. However, aerobic exercise also releases brain chemicals called endorphins, which specifically raise the spirits, combating depression and bringing a sense of euphoria (the so-called 'runner's high'). Other chemicals released in response to regular aerobic activity boost the immune defence system and help us to overcome infectious illnesses and cancerous cell changes.

What is the best way to achieve these benefits?

Isn't it good news that you can gain all these advantages while making minimal changes to your current lifestyle? In fact, it has been proved scientifically that slight increases in activity carried out regularly are, in the long term, safer and more beneficial than lengthy sessions demanding effort.

The study that came to this conclusion, carried out at the Emory University School of Medicine in Georgia, confirmed something we already knew about regular exercise: it protects the body against heart and circulatory disease by increasing the number of cholesterol-fighting molecules in the body (high levels of the unhealthy low-density kind of cholesterol, referred to as LDL, lead to furred-up arteries, heart-attacks and strokes).

However, experiments on participating student volunteers who had just started attending exercise classes showed that short bursts of activity either failed to produce this effect or actually raised the levels of cholesterol.

The researchers concluded that these results would be bad news for the many enthusiasts who adopt a binge and starve approach to exercise. Sampath Parthasarathy commented in the *Journal of the American Heart Association* that 'regular exercise acts like a vaccine on the immune system, reducing the risks of suffering from a heart attack or stroke'.

There was some comfort, however, according to Dr Parthasarathy, for the boom and bust exercisers, who believe that jogging, step classes or a spot of tennis in the summer makes it safe for them to return to their couch potato habits for the rest of the year. Short-term exercise, it appears, helps to shunt cholesterol out of the bloodstream and into the liver, where it can be broken down and therefore does less harm.

We'll look at some painless ways of becoming more active in the next chapter but, first, we have to discover just what constitutes aerobic exercise for each of us.

What is aerobic exercise for you?

This, of course, varies depending how fit you are. Roger Bannister – the first athlete to break the barrier of the four-minute mile – was undoubtedly aerobically challenged by his feat. You and I might be aerobically challenged by a brisk walk up a moderately steep hill. An elderly patient visiting the bathroom unaccompanied for the first time after a couple of weeks in bed, might find the five-minute round trip muscularly very taxing. So, you see, comparing one individual with another is meaningless, which is why, unless you are training for a competitive sport such as running, swimming or squash, you can happily gain health benefits and improve your fitness entirely free of the fear of failure. You cannot be *bad* at aerobic exercise. You either do it and enjoy its benefits or you avoid it and do without them.

Aerobic exercise makes us sweat and pant a little (but not enough to stop us chatting while we're doing it, remember) and it also increases our pulse rate. One of its most vital benefits to us is its strengthening effect on the heart and increased efficiency it brings to its pumping action. However, this cannot be accomplished without physically challenging the heart. When the pulse rate accelerates, the heart is, in fact, responding to the exercised muscles' increased oxygen requirement. Oxygen is needed to release energy from glucose and glycogen in the muscles, just as it is with more familiar fuel – paper, sticks and coal for a fire – when we wish it to burn and release heat energy. The heart, therefore, beats more rapidly to carry the extra oxygen to the needy muscles.

The lungs, in turn, take more frequent breaths, so that we are both inhaling extra oxygen and getting rid of the mounting load of carbon dioxide and other waste products created by the higher fuel consumption. Metabolic waste is also eliminated via the skin in sweat and the kidneys in urine.

So, is it enough just to know that aerobic exercise bumps up our heart rate and makes us breathe harder, but not too hard? No, we can personalize our health goal more accurately than this. Table 1 shows the recommended exercising pulse rates to aim at, according to your age and level of fitness.

When using Table 1 refer to the higher of two ages if you are between them. Most importantly, never aim to reach your maximum heart rate (given in the second column). Exercise to raise your pulse up to the figure in the third column if you are unfit or to the figure in the fourth column if you are fit. These are far from arbitrary figures, by the way – they have been worked out under carefully controlled and scrutinized laboratory conditions by experts studying hundreds of individuals and their responses to aerobic (and anaerobic) exercise.

Table 1: Recommended pulse rates to aim for when exercising by age and level of fitness

Age	Maximum heart rate	Exercising pulse rate if unfit	Exercising pulse rate if fit
16	204	123	164
18	202	122	162
20	200	120	160
22	198	119	158
24	196	118	157
26	194	116	155
28	192	115	154
30	190	114	152
32	188	113	150
34	186	112	149
36	184	110	147
38	182	109	146
40	180	108	144
45	175	105	140
50	170	102	136
55	165	99	132
60	160	96	128
65	155	93	124
70	150	90	120
75	145	87	116
80	140	84	112

The choice is yours

Table 2 (overleaf) shows a list of potentially aerobic activities, together with the energy used up while doing them. The numbers of calories they burn is of secondary importance to us here as this book is about effortless exercise rather than weight loss. They are included because many of us like to be told facts and figures concerning healthy lifestyle changes where these are available.

I say 'potentially aerobic' because, as I have explained previously, the activity has to be sufficiently vigorous to increase your pulse and make you slightly breathless. Gardening, for instance, can consist of sitting on a lawn next to a flower border, occasionally plucking out the odd weed. Doing this would mean you were using up some extra energy compared to sitting still and reading the newspaper, for instance, but you are not challenging your heart and lungs by doing so. It's up to you to make your chosen exercise supply you with the aerobic benefits you seek.

Table 2: Activities and the numbers of calories burned in an hour

Activity	Calories used per hour
Bowling	250
Cleaning windows	350
Cycling	400
Dancing	300
Football	450
Gardening	250
General housework	190
Golf	250
Horse riding	450
Ironing	250
Jogging	500
Mowing the lawn	400
Running	900
Scrubbing floors	275
Skiing	500
Swimming	500
Walking	250

I have included running to provide a reference point against which to compare other activities. However, unless you are already fit – and known how to go about it – I strongly recommend that you stay away from running, jogging and the more physically demanding types of exertion until you are in better shape.

Try something new

You now have the perfect excuse to take up something you have always fancied doing. If you can, choose something interesting, something you will enjoy learning about and make you long to become proficient enough at it to at least enjoy it. If you are an animal lover, have you considered horse riding? It burns up, on average, a respectable 450 calories an hour, meanwhile strengthening and toning your leg, back and abdominal muscles (and other postural muscles you may not yet know you possess). You could take lessons together with a friend or family member – or set aside an hour for your personal enjoyment once or twice a week.

If finances are tight, try another approach (there usually is one!). Many stables are only too glad of an extra pair of hands to help with mucking out the horses' stalls or boxes (forking up soiled wet straw and replacing it with clean). You could have a lesson once a week, say, in lieu of payment. The bonus is that mucking out – like most things – is an aerobic activity in itself. Go easy on the forking at first if you are used only to a little light dusting. The wet straw is not particularly heavy, but the bending and lifting can cause backache if you are unused to it. Stables also smell pleasant (to stable hands, anyway) and cleaning tack and grooming the horses usually afford the opportunity to chat and catch up with local gossip.

Once you are mounted, learning to rise to the trot can be challenging – it is certainly one of the more aerobic aspects of riding when you start. You *will* suffer (a bit) from a sore bottom and inner thigh muscles and will probably feel – and look like – a sack of potatoes in the saddle, but the body adapts surprisingly quickly to new demands made on it – and once you have mastered the art of trotting, like riding a bike, you will never forget it.

Lessons on the lunge rein in an indoor or outdoor school ensure you the personal attention of your instructor and the optimal use of all relevant muscles. Later on, hacking alone or in a group in the countryside or a park, around fields or across moors, is delightfully invigorating, providing plenty of fresh air to blow the cobwebs away. Horse riding also offers the bonus of a closer knowledge of, and friendship with, one of man's best four-legged friends. A fully balanced understanding of, and harmony with, the horse and its movements are primary goals in learning to ride, and experience of this at its best helps to establish inner strength, resilience and tranquillity.

Nella
Nella was 60 when she took up riding.

'I have always loved animals and admired horses from a safe distance – I wasn't too sure I could handle them close up! Then one of my nieces, aged nine, was badly injured in a road accident and later on was offered the opportunity to ride on horseback with

Riding for the Disabled. I sometimes took her to the stables when my sister was busy with the other children, and I was very impressed by the gentle giants whom all the children seemed to love so much. I was a stone (about 6 kg) or so overweight, had moderately raised blood pressure and had always suffered from insomnia. Otherwise I was in good health and my doctor said there was no reason I should not learn.

'I took up riding a year ago, and I just can't tell you the benefits I have gained. It's a release from stress when my husband's been getting on my nerves – he retired several years ago and we are together all day. Consequently I sleep better and, having regained my normal weight, no longer have to take blood pressure tablets, although the doctor is still checking it every three months. I have made lots of friends of all ages and enjoy a nice hack out across the fields three times a week in all weathers. I would recommend it to anyone.'

Jazz it up

If you'd prefer music to set your exercise rhythm rather than a horse, you could try jazz, modern sequence or some other variety of dance class – even belly dancing, which has become increasingly popular in both the UK and Australia over the past five years. Belly dancing is not only liberating and erotic, it provides all the fun of dressing up in exotic dancing gear and Eastern jewellery. It also improves flexibility and muscle tone, and you can make it as aerobically challenging as you wish while learning to perform intricate steps and movements to the haunting Middle Eastern or Indian melodies.

It is now also possible for adults to learn ballet in certain areas, so if you are a fan, this may be the choice for you. Obviously you cannot hope to excel like professionals who started as tots, but this should not be in your mind if you take it up. Barre work, of course, improves stamina, flexibility and muscle tone, posture and physical grace. Dance itself is aerobically challenging and the music accompanying this and any other type of dance can help to relieve stress, tension and depression. (The 'wrong' kind of sound for you can have the opposite effect, so if you decide on dancing be sure to pick a type with music you enjoy.)

Just remember, warming up and cooling down before and after dancing and, indeed, all aerobic classes is very important. Also, go easy with line or tap dancing, which can play havoc with the knees and other weight-bearing joints.

Sue

Sue was 22 when she took up dancing while revising for her final exams at university.

'The run-up to finals sounds a queer time to take up something new, but I needed to get out of the student lodging where I was living and mix with other people. Pop music – which I have always hated – seemed to be on 24 hours a day, and all any of us could talk about was the exam syllabus and whether we thought we would pass. It was driving me nuts . . .

'Anyway, I was in the library and saw an advertisement for sequence dancing. I wasn't too sure what this was, but I felt certain that it would not include pop, heavy metal or rap! I was the youngest in the group of about 15 men and women, but they were delighted at my interest, and took me under their wing. The dance music was really old-fashioned – the kind my gran likes to listen to – but because I was missing her, I found dancing to it very soothing and relaxing. In fact, sequence dancing is so much fun, I forget all about the health benefits of aerobic exercise while I am doing it.'

Take to it like a duck!

For safe exercise, enjoyment, accessibility and economy, it is hard to beat swimming and/or aquarobics. Unless you swim in the sea during the off-season or in a solitary pond, lake or river (many people do), you will have the company of like-minded enthusiasts and often (depending where you decide to go) the added security of qualified instructors and people trained in lifesaving.

The sea (choose somewhere safe!) has the attraction of any natural element and the surroundings are often beautiful (which calms the mind and emotions and releases muscular tension, encouraging the proper use of underexercised muscles). An indoor or outdoor swimming pool, on the other hand, offers current-free swimming in all seasons, is often heated and treated against contaminants. There are also changing rooms and lockers in which to safely stow your belongings.

Best of all, water offers buoyancy, supporting the body and limbs and making them virtually weightless while you are exercising and swimming. This is one of the reasons for its inclusion in both human and animal physiotherapy, and why swimming is so beneficial for people with all sorts of lower limb and back injuries.

The support offered by water also helps to explain the broad appeal of aquarobics in most parts of the world. Best described as a gentle form of aerobics performed standing, walking and/or dancing in a swimming pool, aquarobics is far less daunting for newcomers than land-based aerobics. It is also suitable for people of all ages and abilities. Equally beneficial is the fact that it uses the resistance of the water to enable you to work at your personal aerobic best. Aquarobics doesn't cause you to get up a sweat exactly, because of how it is performed, but it burns up calories and you feel a beautiful glow by the end of the class, which remind you of the health benefits you've just so enjoyably gained.

Carol-Anne

This is the story of Carol-Anne, aged 40.

'I first came across aquarobics when I was visiting our local pool, trying to psych up the courage to start swimming again. I am 5 foot 3 inches (about 1.53 m) tall and, at 14 stone (89 kg), I was hugely overweight (my normal weight being around $8\frac{1}{2}$ stone [54 kg]). Having been through a very stressful year, I had started to binge eat and drink, and my blood pressure had gone sky high. My doctor was adamant about my need to lose weight and urged me to take up some regular exercise.

'I chose swimming because I could already do it and, by going very early in the morning (or mid-afternoon on weekdays, as I thought), I was hoping that I could get in some practice without too many people seeing my ghastly body.

'Catching sight of the women's-only aquarobic class gave me a huge confidence boost. There they all were, about 25 women of all ages and sizes – from painfully thin to more obese than I – and they all looked as though they were enjoying themselves. They were moving about, jumping up and down in time to the rhythm of music played on a ghetto blaster on the pool side, aided and abetted by a very feisty instructor who, I noticed, encouraged everyone in turn and made fun of nobody. I went to the next class and have been weekly ever since. My weight is coming down slowly but surely and I am as pleased as Punch at how much fitter I am (I can go upstairs easily now without practically collapsing at the top).'

Fed up? Just walk out!

Providing you have a reasonably healthy back and legs, there is no simpler nor more suitable exercise than walking. It's free, accessible wherever and whenever and can be customized to suit personal fitness requirements without the need for lessons, help or advice. Walking should appeal to you if you are impatient, easily bored and like to get your exercise for the day truly out of the way. Although, of course, you appreciate its benefits, you really don't want to hang around, buy special gear, change your clothes or go anywhere for exercise sessions.

Walking (as briskly as *you* feel comfortable) is recommended not only by fitness experts and exercise instructors, but also by cardiologists (heart specialists), lung specialists, diabetes experts and other health consultants. It can be done in such a way to suit the tastes and requirements of anyone needing to reduce their weight and recover from a heart attack or long spell in bed. Walking can also minimize the risk factors of an operation such as coronary bypass or open heart surgery if used to improve fitness beforehand.

Being simple and accessible, walking is the activity most likely to get dedicated couch potatoes, overweight fractious children and anyone suffering from anxiety or depression off their backsides and 'up and at it'! So, if at the moment of reading this you still feel rooted to your armchair, 'guilty' about your sedentary lifestyle, but not guilty enough to do anything about it, try this one for size. Stand up, walk to your front door, open it and go outside, then walk for five minutes in any direction. Neither dawdle nor rush, just march off with your chin in the air, so that any onlooker would think: 'I wonder where he/she is going!' Then turn around and walk back.

Congratulations! You are fantastic! You've broken down a mental barrier and have just taken your first step towards aerobic exercise. Do it again tomorrow.

Sheila
Sheila is 51.

'I never, ever in a million years believed I would take up any form of exercise. I am physically lazy by nature – I hated PE and games at school and vowed never to do them again when I left – and although I work very hard mentally at my job, I have always insisted on simply crashing out in the evenings and at weekends. Even my husband's pleas to join him on country rambles at the weekends met with firm refusals. I ate fairly healthily and did not smoke, so I thought I was quite healthy enough . . .

'Then my husband had a heart attack at the age of 53. He seemed so fit and was always the active one. The heart specialist explained that gentle walking was essential for his recovery and asked me to accompany him to keep an eye on him – especially in the early stages. I could hardly say no.

'So, we began taking small walks around the village and, later on, across meadows and fields. I soon began to realize how much I had been missing. It felt so good to use my legs and feet, swing my arms about, take deep breaths and admire the seasons and nature. Roy went from strength to strength, and I am pleased to say that I did, too. I shed the odd 7 to 8 lbs (3 to 3.5 kg) surplus weight I was carrying, and we now go out for longer walks nearly every day. I feel less stressed at work, and I sleep better too.'

Never too old to exercise

According to a report published in *Geriatric Medicine* in May 1986 (the findings of which have been repeated by many studies since), only a fraction of physical decline in strength and stamina in elderly people results from a disease; most of it is caused by underuse. Typically, if we are stiff, weak, in pain or otherwise compromised, at any age, but especially, perhaps, as we get older, we start to make less use of the particular part of the body concerned. This may be the legs, say, after fracturing a hip joint or back after arthritis develops and, consequently, we become less active.

This means that most of us, after a certain age, are less fit and able than we could be, simply because we don't do any exercise. In fact, Oxford Community Physician, Dr J. A. Muir-Gray, pointed out in this report that many older people's (veterans') sporting records demonstrate that the loss of fitness due to age alone is a great deal less than most of us, including doctors, might suppose: 'There is every reason to encourage people to try to keep fit as they grow older as a way of preventing some of the problems typical of old age.' He gave compelling evidence that fitness can be regained in old age. In one study, a seven-week programme reconditioning elderly participants to regular physical exertion improved their capacity for aerobic exercise by 30 per cent, while maximum oxygen intake was brought quickly to the level associated with a sedentary person 10 to 20 years younger than the participants.

Other research studies indicate that suppleness, strength and skill, as well as stamina, can be significantly improved in elderly people. Table 3 appeared in *Geriatric Medicine* in May, 1986, and the fit veterans' peak performance is surprisingly close to that of their younger counterparts (British Veterans' Cycling Records, 1983).

Table 3: Fit male veterans' peak performance

25 miles		50 miles		100 miles	
Age	Time	Age	Time	Age	Time
43	52.45	43	1.47.38	43	3.51.25
66	57.05	66	1.52.41	66	4.16.37
77	1.08.00	77	2.19.57	76	5.16.53
82	1.37.00	78	2.52.38		

As you can see, veteran male cyclists with an average age of 66 took only 4.6 minutes longer to complete 25 miles than men averaging 43 years. Men in the 82-year-old bracket took an hour and 37 minutes to cycle this distance compared to the 52.45 minutes of the 43-year-old men.

Doctors have, in fact, been accused of failing to encourage elderly people to exercise in ways that would benefit their health. Despite the clear advantages of regular exercise in our advancing years, according to Professor Marion McMurdo of the Department of Medicine at the University of Dundee, practitioners have spent too much time in search of reasons for older people not to take exercise and too little in promoting its benefits. In a contribution to the *British Journal of Sports Medicine*, she says that both elderly patients and their GPs are afraid that exercise in old age will harm participants and/or that, since chronic disorders originate during our early years, trying to reverse them is a waste of time.

Regrettably, according to Professor McMurdo, this attitude merely helps to increase disability among older people and encourages spiralling healthcare costs. We need to throw out the unrealistic and discouraging image of high-tech aerobics performed by Lycra-clad teenagers with waist measurements in single figures and 'embrace the concept of health and physical activity – walking, dancing, gardening and playing with the grandchildren'.

Excitingly – again according to Professor McMurdo – 'there is no such thing as the inevitability of decline with old age, or the inability to train elderly muscles.' No pensioner has been injured at the University of Dundee's over-sixties exercise classes, which attract about a thousand people per week. The Professor deplores the fact that many people in hospitals, residential homes, day-care centres and so on are missing out on activity that could improve their health and well-being. She would like to see a radical rethink on this topic in all relevant facilities caring for elderly people: 'A public health approach to an ageing society is long overdue. Elderly people must be informed that regular physical activity is both appropriate and desirable in old age, and the older community should be involved in developing a range of services and facilities to back this up.'

These comments are confirmed by other authorities and research studies, agrees the charity Age Concern. In studies performed in the UK and the USA, training three times a week for three months has been shown to strengthen muscles in the over-seventies, while a regular walking programme for this age group reversed deteriorating lung function and a weights programme doubled leg strength. Age Concern's Director General Sally Greengross emphasizes that 'fitness is not just for the agile. No matter how late in life you start, by gradually increasing the amount of exercise you do you can improve your health and well-being.'

Maureen

Maureen, 79, found exercise helped her when she was recovering from a hip replacement operation.

'I had been waiting for a hip replacement for five years when it was finally done late last year. I have a good heart and lungs and have never smoked, so had no medical problems while recovering, but it had been increasingly hard for me to get about in the years leading up to the op, and my doctor said the muscles of my thighs and calves were wasted.

'Once the surgery was over, though, I had some physiotherapy on the hospital ward and again later at the convalescent home. Then, when I went home, I started to attend a Day Centre two days a week where easy movement classes were held by a specialist teacher who helped us individually to carry out the exercise from which we would most benefit. My legs felt really weak – so much so that I felt unsteady and feared falling – but they were very kind and, after using a zimmer frame for a few weeks, I started to strengthen up.

It really is true what my husband used to say – 'use it or lose it!' I can walk to the shops quite easily now, every day, and can also take my Pekinese for a nice walk in the park every afternoon. To tell you the truth, I feel ten years younger since the hip replacement, and most of this is due to becoming so much more active again.'

A number of residential homes and geriatric wards already have exercise programmes in place to achieve these ends. However, it is worth remembering, if you are getting older, that you cannot do yourself a better turn than to get out there and be more active. If you are lonely, socially isolated and feel 'chance would be a fine thing', look on the noticeboard at your local church or your library or health centre. The latter two, at least, should be able to put you in touch with a group or class to which you can travel by bus or in the car of a friendly neighbour willing to give you a lift.

At the very least, take a walk to a shop you enjoy visiting every day – find one that opens on a Sunday too, and most areas have them now. You do not have to buy anything – the majority of corner shopkeepers are streetwise, friendly folk, only too happy to pass the time of day with sometime customers and welcome the sight of a friendly, smiling face.

2
Getting It Right

You need to be deliberately physically active for at least part of each day in order to access the health benefits of exercise. This can be made effortless by making minor adjustments to your daily routine. We will introduce these changes so gradually that you will barely be aware of them. We will also look at how you go about setting aside some time each week for an activity you enjoy, if you wish. First, here's how to transform both personal treats and daily chores into interesting opportunities for physical action.

Personal treats

These are like mini versions of activities you would like to learn, such as those discussed in the previous chapter, only easier to fit in and even more accessible.

Home and leisure
- Think back to when you were a child. Which activities always had you coming back for more? Choose one and buy the appropriate skipping rope, roller or ice skates, kite, scooter, hula hoop (try children's toy shops or the second-hand column of your local newspaper). Next, earmark ten minutes of any daily leisure hour you would normally spend reading or watching television. Go out into the garden, street or local park and relive happy childhood memories. Remember to wear a helmet or protective knee and elbow pads if you are skating or scootering. When your ten minutes are up, back you come. That's your (exercise) duty done for the day. The chances are you will want to spend longer enjoying this new treat than you thought! Gradually build up the time devoted to it by, say, five minutes a week, until you are regularly practising it for half an hour at a time.
- Go with the kids! Surprise your children, friends' children, nephews, nieces or grandchildren by joining in a game you know you would enjoy. Don't be roped into just anything – if footy in the park or rounders on the rec don't grab you, then dig out your bike or borrow one and join them when they go out. Don't try to

match them – you're most unlikely to be able to cycle up steep hills and, at this stage, shouldn't even try. Half a mile to a sweet shop (try not to indulge just because they are!) should be perfect at first, but you will soon be enjoying the fresh air and exercise and wanting to cycle further.

- Games can provide just as many opportunities for you and your children to exert yourself (and, in some cases, are twice as much fun) as formal pastimes and sports. Depending on their ages, try musical jumps, musical chairs, ring a ring o' roses and friendly wrestling – these are all suitable indoor pursuits.

- Alternatively, you could teach the kids old-fashioned games like tag, kick-the-can, grandmother's footsteps and hopscotch. These involve plenty of jumping and running round, and what you (or your parents) used to play as youngsters, might keep yours enthralled for half an hour at least!

- Add some allure to your exercise at least once a week by including it in a home beauty session or grooming. Put on loose, comfortable clothing and spend 10 minutes (later 20 and so on) walking round the block as briskly as you find comfortable. Once you are back indoors, wash and condition your hair, run a bath, add moisturizing bubbles or three or four drops of lavender essential oil and soak to your heart's content. Read a book or magazine, have some music or the radio on and invest in a padded or inflatable neck rest for bathtime use. Dry yourself with a warm, clean, fluffy towel and, if you are a man, clean and file your fingernails and toenails and do any of the other little personal jobs you rarely find time for. If you are a woman, rub moisturizing cream into every part of your skin, dress and give yourself a pedicure and manicure using your favourite nail varnish. Then sit back with more favourite background music, sipping a Virgin Mary or Pink Pony (see below), feeling gorgeous and highly virtuous.

Virgin Mary
150 ml (5 fl oz) good-quality tomato juice
crushed ice cubes
dash of Worcester sauce, if liked
slither of lemon peel

Shake or stir all the ingredients together, sip slowly and enjoy.

Pink Pony
200–300 ml (7–10 fl oz) diet tonic water
crushed ice
dash of angostura bitters
2 maraschino cherries
slither of lemon peel

Shake or stir the first three ingredients together, then mix in the lemon peel and decorate with the cherries. Lie back and enjoy.

Home and work

- *Housework* Turn on some music and dance around the house while dusting. *Really* let your hair down! Bend and stretch to reach dusty and neglected corners. Reach under the bed for stray shoes and other items. Iron with gusto, but first make sure the ironing board is adjusted correctly for your height or you may end up with a backache.
- *Dog-walking* This provides the perfect chance of a brisk walk, as well as a bonding opportunity with man's (and definitely woman's!) best friend. The former will get you back on the exercise track and the latter will help to normalize your blood pressure – particularly if you pat and stroke the dog before and after walking. Larger, more active types of dogs are usually the best choice if your time is limited because they are faster on their feet, but smaller ones can be cajoled into moving at a respectable pace if you allow them a few minutes to sniff about and get that out of the way before you set off.
- *Shopping* 'Not much chance there for a brisk walk' you may think, remembering the bootload of provisions constituting your weekly shop. Why not stagger the load, though, rather than stagger *about* with it, straining your muscles and joints! Walk to your local shops and buy a different type of goods each day – only as much as you can comfortably carry. Fruit, vegetables, meat from the butcher, wet fish and bread and rolls from the bakery are all tastier and better nutritionally when eaten fresh daily. When you do visit the supermarket, you will find your bill and time gratifyingly reduced.

Office or workplace

- Walk upstairs instead of using the lift (attempt only as many flights as you feel comfortable with). If you have a desk job, get up at least once every hour, stretch and walk a few steps – if only between your workstation and the window. Cut yourself off mentally for a moment from your immediate environment (to avoid becoming stale and stressed) by looking out into the street or over the surroundings into the distance. Take six deep breaths, hold each for a few seconds, then exhale slowly. Remember, every little bit of exercise counts. Remaining stress-free also helps to combat fatigue and encourages you to look forward eagerly to a short walk or cycle ride after work.
- Have a wander round the block when you have a five-minute break and make a point of getting some fresh air with a stroll at lunchtime.
- Park your car further than usual from the office or workplace or get off the tube or bus a few stops earlier and walk the rest of the way.

Essential to the enjoyment of all treats, including those of the exercise variety, are the right time, the right place and the right company.

The right time

By the 'right time' I mean both *when* you are more active and for how *long*.

For goodness sake when?

If you claim that you haven't the time, then you are coming up with the commonest obstacle cited by people in the UK – four out of five of us are exercising too little to improve or maintain our health. This immediately begs the question of how much our health as a nation would improve if we all made time to be more active. You may assert that it is impossible to make the time, yet the real tragedy is that no one can make time wait.

'Use it or lose it' is a fact of life. Every day spent lying in bed, watching TV or surfing the Internet, robs our heart, lungs, bones, joints and muscles of a tiny portion of their strength and vitality and, therefore, of their usefulness to us. Regular, moderately challenging

21

exercise makes us breathe more deeply, utilizing more of our lungs and taking in more oxygen, which benefits the brain and, indeed, in turn the whole of the body. Exercise improves the circulation of blood and lymph, strengthening the immune system and maintaining the health of the coronary arteries, which deliver nutrient- and oxygen-rich blood to the heart. These and other benefits abound, in return for just 30 minutes of extra effort, 5 days a week. This represents only 1.5 per cent of the total time in a week. So what can we mean when we say we can't 'fit exercise in'?

Let's ask ourselves what we do (and always will) find time for. Well, first, there are daily essentials, such as our job, the school run, shopping, walking the dog, paying the bills. Then there are our equally essential leisure pursuits, when we unwind, changing into our oldest clothes, pottering about in the garden or study, reading a book, listening to music and maybe sharing a glass of wine and a meal with friends. For those of us with partners, there is also the shared pleasure of intimate moments when we cuddle, make love and fall asleep in one another's arms.

By making time to care for our bodies and minds with extra exercise, we are helping to ensure our enjoyment of all these other pleasures for many years to come.

How long for?

Scientists studying exercise since the early 1980s have shown that we need to spend 25 to 30 minutes each day of the working week in increased physical activity to ensure health improvements. Do not be daunted by this! You have to remember that you will either be walking at a moderate pace (which is something you do without even thinking about it, anyway) or taking up an activity of your choice that you really enjoy. If you are very overweight, have high blood pressure or any other ongoing health problems or are unsure of your fitness level, ask your doctor's advice on how much exercise you should do before you start.

Even if you are relatively fit (considering your sedentary lifestyle), it's essential to start slowly and build up gradually over a period of weeks until you are easily walking (or whatever) for up to 30 minutes at a time.

The most vital message I can give you at this stage is that *any physical exertion, no matter how small, is much, much better than none.* We live such chronically inactive lifestyles in the West that even the tiniest increase in effort will prove beneficial. You can also expect to notice the difference shortly after starting to build in some regular activity. You will be much more likely to make the change a permanent one – if you plan ahead and find the best time to fit it in.

The right place

Suitable locations depend, naturally, on your choice of activity. If you are a city dweller, then parks and public gardens are great for walking – with or without a dog. If you're lucky enough to live in the country, then you have the choice of lanes, fields and villages, woods, moors and perhaps beaches and lakesides.

If swimming appeals, then the sea and indoor and outdoor pools are all possible choices.

Riding with a good stable or school, you will be taken along park tracks if you live in a town or across meadows or heaths in the country in good weather or under shelter in an indoor school in bad weather.

Dancing of all types is likely to be done in a hall or leisure centre if you join a group. If you dance alone, then you have the whole house in which to perform, with your favourite music on, whenever you have the house to yourself.

Other choices include the house of a friend with whom you have arranged to exercise and your garden, patio or conservatory. You may even be tempted by a quiet retreat, such as a spa or similar, miles from anywhere that offers nurturing TLC and a variety of therapies, including complementary therapies, if you have been unwell or very stressed and are seeking to reclaim your health.

The right person

This really is an extension of the ideas on venues for your exercise, but it is worth considering finding an exercise buddy if you lack motivation – and tend to start things in a fit of enthusiasm and then that enthusiasm rapidly peters out. Many of us feel we might do better were we to share the experience of exercising for health, especially if it is an entirely new venture and we're lacking confidence.

Your partner or another family member might be ideal, providing they take the matter seriously enough to keep at it, and work with you towards mutual goals. This does not mean that you both (or all) have to be at the same stage of fitness – it could be fun and exhilarating walking with a teenage son or daughter, for instance, so long as you each exercise at your own pace.

On the other hand, people are not always sympathetic to other family members' attempts to follow a healthier diet or a fitness plan, so someone you know from work, a neighbour or an acquaintance you make while walking the dog, riding, swimming or whatever may better meet your needs.

Having an exercise buddy is beneficial in several ways. You can motivate one another, set goals to suit mutual requirements and, if you can keep up a conversation while exercising, you can be certain that you are not walking, skating, dancing or whatever at too fast a rate.

Getting results

How soon can you expect to see results from your exercise plan and how can they be measured?

Your body mass index (BMI) and waist to hip ratio are useful general indications of how healthy you are because they reflect whether or not you are overweight more accurately than your weight in kilos or pounds is able to. It is, however, technically possible to be overweight in terms of the BMI scales – that is, have a higher than normal BMI – without having a spare tyre or even a little bit of flab in sight.

Muscle weighs more than fat, so, for this reason, bodybuilders and athletes are exceptions to the rule and frequently weigh much more than others of the same build, sex and height. They are the opposite of obese, of course, but it is easy to see why top sportspeople, bodybuilders and others seem to 'run to fat' when they cease their punishing exercise and training schedules. Their large muscles weaken and reduce in size, then are replaced by layer on layer of adipose tissue, which is fat stored below the surface of the skin. Conversely, there are also apparently skinny people with low BMIs who, for their build, size and height, are actually obese because they are carrying around an excess of fat.

Your BMI can be calculated by dividing your weight in kilograms by your height in metres squared (or by multiplying your weight in pounds by 700 and dividing the result by your height in inches squared). For example, the calculation for someone weighing 80 kg (176 lbs) and standing 1.60 m (63 in) tall would be:

$$\frac{80}{1.60} \times 1.60 = 31.2$$

(in imperial measures that would be:

$$176 \times \frac{700}{63 \times 63} = 31.1)$$

Table 4 shows BMI ranges and the categories they relate to for your reference.

Table 4: Body mass indices and categories
they relate to

Category	BMI
Underweight	below 19
Normal	20–25
Overweight	26–30
Obese	over 30
Morbidly obese	over 40

For the morbidly obese, drastic measures need to be taken to avoid the very real threat of early death.

The BMI categories and scale were orginally formulated by the US Department of Agriculture and Health and Human Services which, in 1995, published new healthy weight ranges for adult men and women. The ranges, proposed by a panel of experts, are based on a detailed review of the literature and case studies dealing with weight-linked disease and death risks over a range of BMI values. The upper limit of healthy weight sits at a BMI level of around 25, based on the significant increase in the ill effects of obesity among people with BMIs above this cut-off point. The lower boundary of healthy weight is a BMI of 19, although no one is certain whether or not there are health risks if you are underweight to this degree. Risks of disease and early death increase significantly for BMI values between 28 and 29, which is the dividing line between being moderately and severely overweight.

Like the BMI, the waist to hip ratio (WHR) was derived from a research study looking at links between obesity, heart disease and diabetes – this time carried out in Canada. The accumulation of fat over the tummy area (known clinically as abdominal adiposity) can be assessed from a person's WHR or from their waist circumference alone. Research suggests that either measurement may be a more accurate predictor of an increased risk of early death from being overweight than the assessment of general excess body fat. Health experts find WHR particularly relevant for assessing patients who combine a weight that is borderline high with a personal or family medical history of an increased health risk.

To find your WHR, stand up, breathe in deeply then exhale. Now measure your girth at the level of your navel (or the level at which your tummy sticks out most, whichever is the greater) then your hips, at the level at which your bottom projects most. Keep the tapemeasure in close contact with the skin but without indenting it at any point. Divide the first of your readings by the second, thus:

$$\frac{\text{Abdominal circumference}}{\text{Hip circumference}}$$

WHR values above 1.0 for men and above 0.8 for women are associated with an increased risk of diabetes, hypertension (raised blood pressure), stroke, coronary heart disease and early death from all causes. A waist measurement alone in excess of 100 cm (39 in) in either sex has similar health risk implications. As you are no doubt aware, most overweight people fall into one of two categories – ample apples or portly pears. Ample apples are so-called because they have a more spherical outline, storing a fair proportion of their adipose tissue (fat surplus) around their middles. Portly pears (remember 'pear-shaped' is commonly a term for things going wrong as well as the hated 'typical' overweight British body shape) are, by comparison more hourglass-shaped, storing more weight around the hips and bottom than anywhere else. You may be safer as a pear than an apple, but both shapes carry health risks that can be greatly reduced by regular exercise.

Alternatively, the amount of fat being stored can be assessed by using special callipers available from most good pharmacies. Callipers are inexpensive and should come with a chart indicating healthy and unhealthy fat folds at various points on the body. Their disadvantages are a tendency to pinch the skin and the need to involve someone else in the measurement, for instance when applying them between the shoulder blades. You can also calculate and monitor personal fat levels (which, by the way, I regard as a highly personal matter!) using a custom-designed body fat machine. You need to enter details of your gender, weight, height and how athletic you are to obtain an accurate reading.

Mary

Mary, 35, PA to a politician, thought she couldn't possibly fit exercise into her schedule.

'I had realized for ages that I wasn't active enough to be healthy, but despaired of ever being able to fit in the time to exercise properly. By this, I meant going to a gym (horrid thought!), running for half an hour several times a week or swimming 20 lengths of our local pool. Then I accepted an offer in a national newspaper for a health assessment at a local private health clinic and was appalled by their findings and predictions of my future health trend.

'I knew I was overweight – I have always been on the heavy side and, because my partner loves me however I look, I had no motivation for making changes. But tests at the clinic revealed that I had a BMI of 31, and a WHR of 1.1. They told me that I had an increased risk of death from coronary heart disease and stroke, as well as diabetes and cancer. My father died from diabetic complications and I had been shown to be a borderline diabetic during my pregnancy when expecting our daughter. My mother had breast cancer at the time (she is now very well, thanks to treatment) and I certainly did not want to follow in either of my parents' footsteps.

'I started walking a little longer each day – leaving my car at the far end of the car park, walking instead of driving to the shops and plodding up the five flights of stairs at work. It all seemed very difficult at first, but I soon noticed that I was getting far less out of breath than previously, and this gave me heart. My daughter was pretty overweight too, and we decided to exercise together – walking our dog a bit further every day, swimming once a week in the sea very near our house, and we even bought a secondhand exercise bike to tot up the miles.

'I changed my diet a bit – fewer sweets between meals and fruit or yogurt for pudding – but I had never really overeaten. As soon as I saw the pounds rolling off (my daughter found the same), I got really enthusiastic and began to exercise a little daily.

I now have a BMI of 25 and a WHR of 0.7. I know from this that I have defeated the trend I was on towards an early death from excess fat but, more importantly, I feel by comparison a million dollars. My husband is so impressed, that he has started to exercise several times weekly too. Now the three of us go out together, increasing our weekly activity levels and feeling far, far better for our effort.'

Caroline
Caroline, 43, housewife and mother of three, has this to say about exercise.

'I have never been overweight – underweight, if anything – but when I reached my thirties, I found that little bits of exertion, like climbing the stairs at home, running for a bus and carrying shopping home from the supermarket, were making me very tired. I had never consciously exercised, but I suppose I believed that looking after three children under ten and a husband more than compensated in the health stakes.

'I went to my doctor and he prescribed iron tablets because my periods were heavy, but they had no effect. Then I read a magazine article about exhaustion resulting from stress and daily wear-and-tear and how some fresh air and exercise might be the key to putting things to rights. I started taking short, ten-minute walks every morning and, to my surprise, I felt and slept better than I had for years.

'Then my husband decided to buy the kids a dog! I wasn't keen but, like the rest of the family, I very soon grew to love him and took him out every afternoon across the fields near where we live. He was very active, being a West Highland White Terrier, and soon I was looking forward to our daily outing of 45 minutes or more – forgetting meanwhile about my determination to exercise more.

'You could say that exercise crept up on me silently, in the form of our dear Pip. He was ill for five days with a canine virus and, besides the worry, I really missed our daily outings. When he recovered, he and I went off across the fields just as before, and I started to run and race with him over the sand dunes, in celebration of his return to life. The children were ecstatic that Pip recovered and now we all go out at least five times a week, running and playing with Pip, and walking him around the streets for his shorter evening and early morning walks. I could swear that the deeper breaths of oxygen we all take and the yards we all run keeping up with our dear dog have added years to all our lives.'

3

Stretching Exercise

Writers of fiction sometimes describe cats (and women) as 'stretching luxuriously'. Perhaps this is simply cliché, but think back to the last time you were squashed into a cramped, confined space – this morning? Right now? On a bus or train in London, in a busy lift, a crowded sports stadium, or the back of a small car? You will undoubtedly remember how the *need* to stretch soon becomes obsessional, and how, once released from your torture, inhaling deeply and reaching out in all directions, extending those cramped muscles, feels like heaven.

Apart from providing delicious freedom and release, regular stretching is a vital part of effortless exercise. It unknots those muscles most prone to the effects of tension, such as in the scalp and neck, shoulders, upper and lower back, face and jaw. Related ailments stretching can relieve include tension headaches and migraine, digestive disorders, high blood pressure, urinary incontinence, PMS and period pain, and insomnia. Stress-related complaints related to poor posture include a stiff neck, aching shoulders, neuralgia (nerve pain) of the arms and legs and, of course, backache.

Before we look further at the benefits of particular sorts of stretching, here are some simple exercises you can do at odd moments throughout the day, when the need arises. They can improve your quality of life, just as they have for the people whose stories are included below.

On waking

Stretch and wriggle freely in bed, stretching body areas gently and randomly in every direction. Stretch arm, leg, tummy and back muscles gently while you are still relaxed and warm. Do this lying face down and face up until your muscles feel satisfied.

Sharon
Sharon is aged 20.

'I had been seeing doctors since I was in my early teens for an aching lower back. I can't remember ever having injured my spine but, from the age of 12 onwards, I found it difficult to keep going all day because pain would start at the back of my pelvis and I'd need to sit down and rest. Mum took me to our GP and I had X-rays, scans and blood tests. All they could come up with was that my lower three lumbar vertebrae had oversized bony projections at the back and that these might be pressing on soft tissue from time to time, causing inflammation. The swollen tissues in turn pressed on pain-sensitive nerves and the whole of my lower back often felt like it was on fire with pain.

'I had a lot of time off from school that first year, especially before and during my periods because the back pain seemed to aggravate the bloated feeling and cramp. I would end up in bed with a paracetamol and a hot water bottle. I got very fed up with this, though, because I wanted to pass my school exams and I was missing out on my social life with school friends. Then Mum took me to a physiotherapist a friend recommended and she gave me some wonderful advice. She asked if I knew the slogan about backache – 'never take a backache lying down'. I didn't, but Mary explained that hours of unnecessary rest weakened the belt of muscles around our tummies and backs that acts like a corset, keeping our organs and spinal bones in place.

'To strengthen my lower back, she told me to wriggle down the bed several times every day, lying on my back and reaching down as far as possible, first with one leg and then with the other – it's a bit like marching on the spot except you are lying down. It really wiggles your hips and frees stiff areas that have become hard to mobilize. If you do it properly, you can wriggle your way right down the bed (without using your hands or arms) and this helps to release pressure on soft tissue around the spine.

'I've done this faithfully every morning and night and occasionally in the middle of the day, ever since. My back still aches at times, but I can do practically everything I want, including swimming and playing tennis, although I do not do hard impact sports such as squash any more.

'Mary also taught me a useful stretch exercise to relieve pain in my back if the nerves do get irritated. I lie on my back on my bed (without a pillow) and bring my knees up to my chest. Then I clasp my knees in my arms and rock gently back and forth once or twice, along the line of my body. Finally, once my back has got used to this, I join my hands in front of my bent knees, and gently squeeze my legs in their grasp, while raising my head a few inches from the bed surface. This stretches the spine all along its length, increasing the spaces between the vertebrae where the spinal nerves come out and, in the case of my lumbar region, relieving pain-triggering pressure. Doing this efficently for up to ten minutes a time can often 'switch off' the nagging pain of neuralgia or a trapped nerve and often I can get away without having to take a painkiller.'

Try this treat

If you love seafood, buy some green-lipped mussels for a weekly feast to combat painful joint and soft tissue inflammation. They contain a powerful anti-inflammatory painkiller proven in scientific studies to benefit such conditions. If you aren't a mussel fan, soothe tight muscles with a few drops of the natural muscular relaxant chamomile oil. Add it to your bath water or to a plain carrier oil, such as sunflower or sweet almond, and gently massage it into and around the muscles concerned.

Give yourself a break

When driving, take a break at least hourly. Do the same whenever you are in any other sedentary occupation, especially slaving for hours over a hot computer screen. Get up when at work or at home, stretch your legs, flex your biceps and forearm muscles, stretch your neck and shoulders, reach for the sky and bend over gently as far as you comfortably can. This flexes and extends your whole spine. Go outside to do this wherever feasible, adding a few extra steps and some fresh air to your daily activity programme.

Paul

Paul is 54.

'I was a drugs rep for years and had to visit a number of GP medical practices every day, five days a week. This could mean driving up to 200 miles or more daily, as well, of course, as humping all my demonstration equipment, laptop, samples and paperwork in and out of the car at every healthcentre I visited.

'I had played football to league standard until I was in my late twenties and suffered a number of back strains and falls because I always played goalkeeper. My back started to become troublesome about five years after I started repping. I went to my doctor, but he just prodded and poked around, said it was my job and prescribed a non-steroidal anti-inflammatory drug similar to, but stronger than, Nurofen. It helped a bit, but I had to stop taking it when I developed a hiatus hernia and my stomach became sick and inflamed with the tablets.

'Finally the job became too stressful and I opted for what I thought would be a quieter life, even if it meant a lower salary. I took my HGV licence and started to drive lorries backwards and forwards between the North of England and the Continent. There was less stress in that my time was more my own and I was not responsible for loading or unloading the goods – just for getting them from A to B. However, I wasn't that much better off, because I still had to keep to a timetable and, when sea crossings were delayed, for instance, due to poor weather conditions, I'd have my work cut out – here or in France or Germany, wherever – to pick up and deliver on time. It often meant breaking the rules and driving for far longer than I legally should – often for ten to eleven hours at a stretch.

'By this time, my back was giving me real gyp – I could hardly walk for the pain when I finally staggered out of the cab at my destination. I was also suffering from heartburn – whatever I ate while working seemed to play me up. In the end I went to see a quack in Belgium who gave me some strong painkillers and urged me to take breaks at at least two-hourly intervals. He also said standing and walking about outside the lorry might help relieve my indigestion as I could be sitting at an angle that cramped my stomach.

'Of course, I was dead against all this at first, because I did not want my money docked for late arrivals, but it was either take his advice or give up. The job suited me in other ways – I still do it, in fact – and now I never drive for more than four hours at the outside – and do try to keep to Dr A's advice of 120 minutes in the driving seat followed by 15 walking about, getting some fresh air and drinking some water.

'I hardly ever have to take painkillers for my back now and haven't had heartburn for over a year.'

Try these treats
Soak in a warm bath at the end of a hectic day when your muscles are weary and add a few drops of marjoram or rosemary essential oils, or a couple of handfuls of the fresh herbs, to the water to encourage tense, irritated muscles to relax.

Soothe heartburn with a cooling, protein-rich, low-fat drink. To 0.5 litre (1 pint) of milk, add a little brown sugar, a newly laid (if possible) free-range egg and a few drops of organic (if possible) almond or vanilla extract to taste if desired. Blend or shake with ice cubes for a creamy consistency and store in vacuum flask for use when travelling or at work. Substitute a mashed banana for the raw egg if you are pregnant, elderly or susceptible to stomach bugs.

Be kind to your spine

When sitting down in the office or at home for long periods, sit up straight and s-t-r-e-t-c-h, with your bottom at the back of the seat and supported by the chair's back. Stretch up and reposition yourself every few minutes, while keeping your back muscles as relaxed as possible. This intermittent stretching and gentle repositioning relieves muscular tension and distributes your weight evenly along the length of your backbone. Sitting too far forwards and leaning at an angle holds the spine at unnatural angles and increases wear and tear in the muscles, joints and ligaments.

Wendy
Wendy is 40.

'I was a reluctant exerciser until I started to suffer from back and neck problems and my GP sent me to a physiotherapist. The first thing he asked me after checking my case history was what kind of exercise I did, for how long at a time and how often. I had to confess that, although I was pretty busy on the home front, looking after my brother's three small children every weekend and writing at home on weekdays, I never actually took exercise as such. He immediately recommended that I go swimming at least twice a week and he also checked my spine for alignment when I was sitting at my computer. He demonstrated, using a model spine and pictures, how my backbone should look, and I had to say that I had probably been mistreating it appallingly!

'My monitor screen had always been rather dark and I had got used to poking my head forwards in order to see properly. I had adapted to technology, as Peter my physio pointed out, instead of adapting technology to my needs! I soon replaced my monitor and, after adjusting my office chair unsuccessfully to various heights, I replaced it with an ergonomically designed typing 'stool'. This is a wooden frame with a seat that positions your pelvis at the natural, anatomically correct angle, and a padded kneeler below and in front, at the correct height and distance to maintain your spine in alignment.

'It felt odd for the first week or so, but I soon got used to it and my neck and shoulder and midback pain have improved beyond recognition, helped especially by stretching upwards and repositioning my spine every few minutes. I do this while working on my stool and also when sitting in ordinary chairs, which I make sure fully support my lower back. Apparently, sitting in the correct position and gentle stretching help to align your vertebrae and their muscles, nerves and blood vessels, so that they receive plenty of oxygen and nutrients and drain away their waste material. Pressure is distributed, too, to the areas where it is meant to be, and the muscles are naturally elongated and exercised by minute, frequent changes in posture.

'Of course, you do need proper exercise as well, especially if you type as many hours a week as I do, but my swimming has taken care of that for me and has helped to strengthen my back.'

Try this treat

To overcome muscle fatigue and recharge your batteries after sitting still and concentrating for ages, play some favourite, really enlivening music that makes you sit up and listen and your pulse beat a little faster. You can stretch your muscles all over, gently, while listening and feel refreshed and invigorated at the end of your ten-minute break.

Contract your tummy muscles

Do this regularly when sitting down or standing for a spell. Like the squeeze-and-stretch manoeuvre recommended to help relieve incontinence by strengthening the pelvic floor, you can do these abdominal squeezes anywhere, at any time, without those around you suspecting a thing. For improved bladder control, squeeze the muscles you normally use when halting a flow of urine midstream. You can practise while actually passing urine to remind yourself where these are, then repeat it while sitting or standing at other times for maximum effect.

Sarah

Sarah is 65.

'I seemed to sag in all directions from my waist downwards, after I went through the change at 55. I did not put on weight, but my muscle tone all seemed to go and I bulged in front like I was six months pregnant. My niece suggested I try something she called ab crunches. She showed me how, by lying on the floor with her knees raised, then clasping her knees and jerking or pulling herself up into a sitting position. She did this about 20 times and said it would help me regain my figure. But it looked very hard and required a lot of effort – to be honest, I was scared of putting something out!

'When I saw my doctor for an annual check, she recommended hormone replacement therapy (HRT) and told me I was wise not to have tried my niece's exercise. Instead, she recommended that I pull my tummy wall in gently while breathing in – sort of back into my abdomen, not upwards into my diaphragm and ribs. This stretches and gently squeezes the muscles, and I hold them squeezed for a count of five, then relax and let them stretch out again as I breathe out. She said I should do this nine to ten times a go, perhaps four or five times a day. At first not a lot happened, as my tummy muscles had become so weak and floppy, but as I persisted, I started to feel them stretching and flexing again, and now, six months later, I have lost a lot of my ugly bulge.

'Mentioning diaphragms, I had been fitted with one a year before I saw my doctor (by my previous GP before I moved house) because I had a bit of trouble passing small dribbles of urine if I laughed or coughed, but my new lady doctor also explained about stretching my pelvic floor muscles to tighten the valve in the pelvic floor that controls urine flow and told me to practise this in runs of ten, also four to five times a day. I did so for three months, then, instead of having my diaphragm checked and replaced, I had it removed altogether to see how I got on.

'I was thrilled that I no longer needed it. I never let my bladder get too full, mind you, but I can laugh or cough or lift up shopping bags without wetting myself. Best of all, the exercise (which I shall continue with indefinitely) has improved our lovemaking as it has helped to tighten the muscles surrounding my vagina. My husband is as pleased with the results as I am!'

Try this treat
Get your partner to massage you before lovemaking with some warm almond oil to which you have added a few drops of essential oil of rose or ylang-ylang, both of which are reported to have aphrodisiac properties.

When you have been sitting

When you are typing, studying books on a table in front of you, sitting down to draw or paint and so on, stand up every half hour or so and take two or three deep slow breaths. Gently roll your head around in a circle, not straining or forcing at all, so your head travels from the chin-on-chest position to looking over your right shoulder, then round and up, smoothly, until you are gazing at the ceiling or sky. Hold this position for a second or two, then look as far to your left as you can without straining. Finally move your head in a smooth arc until your chin is once again on your chest. Repeat three or four times, alternating the direction. This stretches your neck muscles and vertebrae, relieving posture-related headaches and neck stiffness.

Laura
Laura is 32.
'I am an illustrator of technical books and have always worked sitting at my desk rather than in front of a board or easel. I do stare down for quite long periods without moving, usually when choosing colours and seeing how they go together or when simply lost in thought. Then, I guess, my head is held in two different positions – looking at the paper and looking a little beyond the paper at my palette. Anyway, the net result is a lot of tension in my neck and frequently a tension headache after several long days spent in continuous work of this kind.

'I started going for a weekly Indian head massage, which didn't do a lot to help, but then I mentioned my problem to my aromatherapist, Avril, from whom I buy the essential oils I burn while working. They really calm and energize me and help me to think. She suggested that I burn some lavender oil as this is not only calming, but also helps ease muscle soreness. She also gave me upper back and shoulder massages. Using chamomile essence on one occasion and clary sage on another, when my muscles were desperately tight, she kneaded and gently stretched my stressed-out shoulder and neck muscles. Avril also massaged the back of my scalp, where nodules she could feel an inch or so above the hairline were very tender.

'The most important help Avril gave me, though, was to advise me to practise freeing and stretching my neck muscles at least every two hours. I was also to massage my scalp halfway through a working day and at the end of the day before showering. I had been getting bad headaches for some time and the doctor had not been able to find a cause. I believe, as Avril does, that my stiffness and bad heads were both due to poor posture. Muscular stretching has given my work a new lease of life.'

Try this treat
To relieve a persistent headache, make a cold compress for your forehead using very cold water to which you have added a few drops of lavender or peppermint essential oils. Replace compresses as soon as they start to warm up. Mix a couple of drops of your chosen essential oil in about a teaspoon of a carrier oil (available where essential oils are sold), then massage a little of the oil into your temples and/or put a drop or two of an essential oil on a tissue and keep it in your bra or jacket pocket to benefit from the aroma all day.

Oil of marjoram dilates blood vessels and has a warming effect, so can relieve migraine, thought to be triggered by spasm in blood vessels supplying the brain. Use hot compresses in this instance, replacing with fresh as soon as the heat is lost. Some migraine sufferers benefit from sitting under a hairdryer hood during an attack, which similarly dilates the constricted vessels.

Roll your shoulders

Roll them around in as complete a circle as they can comfortably manage. Start by hunching your shoulders up as though trying to touch your ears with them. Then roll them slowly backwards and, when they have travelled as far as they comfortably can, press your elbows inwards behind you as though trying to make them meet. Hold for a few seconds, then bring your shoulders and arms up and forwards until your palms meet in the prayer position, one palm held flat against the other. Do this once or twice, then repeat in the reverse direction.

Peter
Peter is 41.

'I started to feel very tired at work after the air conditioner plant broke down. I also had difficulty remaining awake during meetings, often felt fizzy and had pains in my neck and shoulders. My GP sent me for an X-ray, which showed spondylitis in my cervical spine (small bony protrusions grow out of the vertebrae and press on adjoining soft tissue and spinal nerves). He said there was little that could be done, but that I should keep the upper part of my spine as mobile as possible. It seems that in straining to stay awake and when in pain, I had been hunching my shoulders more than usual (and I am already pretty round-shouldered).

'My father had neck trouble and I remembered him rolling his shoulders around several times a day to gain relief – also circling his head and neck [as described above]. I started to do this and the stretching of my shoulder and upper back muscles felt sensational – I had been bent and cramped for ages, unnecessarily. Extra activity every hour on the hour – which meant getting up and walking a few steps as well as stretching my upper back and neck – gave me more energy. My doctor thinks it is partly because the stretching encourages the blood flow to the brain, neck muscles and joints. Whatever the explanation, I feel better, can stay awake (helped, I am sure, by five-minute breaks at work outside in the open air) and the shoulder and neck pains have improved. I actually feel ten years younger!'

Try this treat
Spices you may well have in your kitchen can give you a glow, raise your spirits and help relieve muscle and joint pain. Make yourself a hot toddy of real ale, to which you add a good grind of nutmeg, a couple of cloves with their heads bashed, a sliver of lemon peel and, perhaps, a stick of cinnamon. If you do not like real ale, try mulled red wine instead, made in the same way.

Relieve face and mouth tension

Screw your face up into an unholy grimace, trying to look as ghastly as possible. Then, stretch each muscle group in turn. Frown hard, feeling your forehead knotting into the typical furrows of an angry frown. Screw your eyes up tightly, hold and relax. Then bunch up your cheeks until they are starting to squeeze your eyes shut. Relax these muscles then purse your lips firmly. Grin as hard as you can, relax, then pretend you are sucking a drink up a very narrow straw – suck for all you're worth!

Finally, bite your teeth together really hard, making your jaw muscles bulge, then relax and concentrate on your tongue. Poke it out as far as you can without hurting, then touch the front, sides and towards the back of your mouth with it, before letting it go completely limp and loose. This exercise is often used as the final stage of muscular relaxation, work on the jaw muscles and tongue being vital preliminaries to an overall state of muscular recovery.

Charlotte
Charlotte, 29, has this to say.

'I had high blood pressure and my doctor prescribed tablets, and also recommended that I try relaxation classes. I did for a bit, then bought a tape and thought I could do it just as well at home myself.

'This was true up to a point, but I never really seemed to relax all over. Just when I thought I was, I would find tension in one or other group of muscles, especially in my jaw. The teacher at the class had told us to relax our tongues, but did not explain that we should stretch them thoroughly first, so that we could fully compare a feeling of tension in the tongue with its opposite. Then I read a magazine article about the tongue being the most essential, if smallest, muscle to let go of, if you want to achieve true relaxation. It described how one should poke it out, circle it around and really stretch it without straining or hurting it.

'I started doing this and everything fell into place. My relaxation took off properly, I took up meditation because I wanted to get as far with relaxation as I could and my doctor has been able to halve the dose of the blood pressure medication I was taking.'

Try this treat
A sore, inflamed tongue is very difficult to relax and will hurt when stretched. Choose a herbal toothpaste – as little as 0.1 per cent of thyme essence in toothpaste will quell oral bacteria, keep the mouth healthy and ulcers at bay. Alternatively, make a fresh-

tasting mouthwash that you can use warm or chilled. Add a pinch of dried thyme or a tablespoon of fresh, to a large cup of boiling water, leave to stew for ten minutes, then strain and use or leave to cool and chill in the fridge.

A little oil of clove or tincture of myrrh applied to the affected area works wonders for toothache and mouth ulcers.

4

Regularizing Your Stretches

In addition to the mini-stretches described in the last chapter, there are more formal effortless exercise systems you can follow on a regular basis, if you wish. These will prolong and intensify the pleasures of stretching for you and maximize its many health benefits.

Systems such as yoga, Pilates and martial arts-related exercises such as t'ai chi and kando, firm and trim the figure and strengthen our 'core' muscles. These are the muscles of the back and the deeper layers of the abdominal wall, which form a supportive and protective corset around the trunk and play a major role in maintaining posture. (Poor posture places unnecessary stresses on the spine, weight-bearing joints and limbs, causing damage and fatigue.) Stretching, in fact, is now known to be highly important for healthy, properly functioning muscles, both when performing mechanical work and at rest. It is comforting to know that caring for our core muscles can take some of the pain out of such activities as digging, laying bricks, vacuuming, carrying shopping and hoisting baby buggies on and off buses or into the boot of the car.

It is because of their unique position, connecting the body's upper and lower halves, that core muscles respond to stretch routines and attempts to improve our posture by working more efficiently. This has a knock-on effect, encouraging other muscles to do the same. We reap the benefits – tiring less easily and relaxing more thoroughly after exercising or a day's work.

Fitness and dance instructors, osteopaths, chiropractors and physiotherapists are now stressing the importance of core stability – that is, stable, naturally balanced core muscles – especially its role in keeping the spine aligned correctly with the rest of the body. To work to maximum effect within the framework of its design – that is, without becoming unhealthily stressed or causing fatigue and pain – the spinal column needs to be straight throughout its length. This means that, from the base of the coccyx, or tail bone, up to the topmost two cervical vertebrae (in the neck) bearing the base of the skull – allowing, of course, for the natural curve at the waist and shoulder – the spine should be straight and not twisted for long periods. The limbs and the upper and lower back must rest or move freely and naturally – never held stiffly or unnaturally so as to overtax one set of muscles at the expense of others. The shoulders and hips also should remain relaxed and evenly poised, for optimal power and action. It is possible to achieve all this *only* if you strengthen and tone the body's muscular core.

Desirable outline

Improving core strength and stability is especially important to dedicated couch potatoes who, as we all know, prefer lounging and sprawling to walking and being active any day of the week. Prolonged sitting over the years, added to the effects of pregnancy and/or becoming obese, pulls the abdominal muscles out of shape, destroying their elasticity and tautness like overstretched elastic bands. It's not surprising that they slacken and sag, robbing the lower spine of its vital support. This not only ruins our outline, it also paves the way to developing inguinal (groin) hernias in men and a prolapsed womb or bladder (and incontinence) in women.

The familiar stomach crunch apparently does nothing for core stability and can have no lasting effect in terms of moulding the front of the tummy into a desirable six-pack. To improve muscle tone in this area really does mean getting back to basics, spending a little while, whenever possible, working gently on our back and abdominal muscles. Hopefully, in this way, we will help ourselves to banish exhaustion, backache, sciatica, aching shoulders, neck pain and posture-related headaches. It doesn't take long, having started regular core stretches, for planned and unplanned physical activities – from a game of beach cricket to professional soccer, making the beds and ironing to loading up the supermarket trolley – to become less of a chore and perhaps even pleasurable.

Stretching the great muscles of the trunk is not only tough on backache and tough on the causes of backache, it also peps up the circulation of blood and lymph and improves the functioning of the heart and lungs (supplementing the benefits of aerobic exercise). As an extension, the kidneys, liver and digestive organs also work better. Further benefits, given time, include a visibly clearer complexion and retarded wrinkling and ageing (due to improved blood circulation to the skin and better functioning of the kidneys and so on), finer coordination and balance and, slowly but surely, the remoulding of a lumpy silhouette into a more desirable, flatter-stomached outline.

Reduction in the risk of injury

With regular exercises that strengthen the core muscles, our everyday movements become less risky mechanically – that is, they are less inclined to result in muscular or spinal injury. How we sit, stand, lift things, even walk, can have a therapeutic effect on body, mind and spirit. Most of us, of course, ignore this, but to our peril. Unaware or heedless of the gathering storm, we place huge demands on our spines daily, only too often under impossible conditions. After, say, hours, days or weeks of inactivity, slouching, sprawling and lying about (when work and other demands permit), and without any warming up beforehand, we lift heavy weights without bending our knees, tug and wrench at immovable furniture, sprint down the road, stagger about with unevenly distributed shopping bags and queue for hours in unsuitable shoes with our hips and spines out of kilter.

Nor were our necks, another postural black spot, designed to be held rigidly for hours, while we drive, sit in front of computers, study or watch TV. Misuse of the cervical (neck) vertebrae, coupled with age-related degeneration, encourages the development of spondylitis (see page 39). Fibrositis, neuralgia (nerve pain) in the upper or lower arm or hand, numbness, tingling, throbbing at night and at rest are all common symptoms. Most of these can be avoided or partially relieved by regular routines to strengthen our core muscles.

Mavis
Mavis is 64.

'When I was at school we did PE and I could always touch the floor without bending my knees. We all enjoyed what we called "physical jerks" and sometimes did it to band music on the wireless, but, like many of my friends, I gave all that up when I left school at 15. Apart from going dancing occasionally while Dan, my husband, and I were courting, I have never done any exercise at all.

'I didn't put much weight on when I was expecting our daughter, nor when I went through the change, but I started to get a very stiff neck, especially in the mornings and in cold winter weather. I thought it was my age, so I put up with it, but then, two years ago, the headaches started and I had to go to see my doctor. I also told him about the shooting pains I was getting in my right arm below the elbow, running down into my hand. They'd keep me awake night after night and, when I also discovered a numb patch on my left hand, I felt sick with fear. One of my aunts, my mother's sister, developed numb patches when she began suffering from multiple sclerosis (MS) and I began to imagine that the same thing was happening to me.

'The doctor put me right about MS – apparently it only affects much younger folk – but he looked at the way I was standing and sitting, measured my height and weight and pressed along the length of my spine. He soon discovered very tender areas to the left of my upper spine, going up into my neck. Being very thorough, he then examined my reflexes and drew round my numb area with a biro after testing it with a sterile needle. He told me the shooting pains and numbness were almost certainly caused by spondylitis in my upper spine, and this was confirmed by X-rays for which he sent me.

'The little tender areas in my upper back were due to local tissue becoming inflamed around small spikes of bone that grow out of the vertebrae in this region, due to both degeneration and the stresses of bad posture. I have always been round-shouldered and walked with a stoop. The inflamed tissue swelling, in turn, pressed on adjacent spinal nerves where they come out between the vertebrae. This gave rise to the headaches, stiff necks and neuralgia, or nerve pain, and numbness in my arms and hands.

'The doctor referred me to a physiotherapist, who gave me some very gentle massage and manipulation and showed me some simple exercises which he said would improve my posture and strengthen the muscles around my upper trunk. He also showed me some simple yoga poses he said would help me. Six months later, I am far less round-shouldered and my neck and head pains have long gone. I know my overall posture has improved because people remark that I look much taller, when most of us lose height with age! I do the stretch exercises every day. My arms and hands are better, but I may never regain full sensation in the numb area due to permanent nerve damage.'

Strong to the core

Most core stability exercises concentrate on the major abdominal muscles, the most prominent of which is the rectus abdominis passing down the front of the abdomen. When the muscles are weak, our stomachs sag; when they are strong and toned, our stomach contours are flat and honed.

The internal and external oblique muscles provide support and shape to the area just above the hips on each side, close to the waist. The transversus abdominis (the fibres of which run across each side of the abdomen to meet in the middle) is vital to posture and should be exercised in any stretching regimen. When weak, it gives a person that dreaded forward bulge from which many women suffer after one (or more often two or more) pregnancies, even if they are not especially overweight.

Equally important to core strength are the erectae spinae (spinal erector) muscles and others that provide stability to the backbone and its muscles, tendons and ligaments. Yoga, Pilates, t'ai chi and related forms of exercise target all the core muscles and others in the rest of the body.

Yoga

Yoga may still have a New Age ring to it, more than 40 years after it was reintroduced into Western society during the 1960s, but you can take or leave the meditation aspect of it as you choose. It is accessible, cheap or free to practise, beneficial to body, mind and spirit and suitable for people of all ages and abilities. It originated as a personal development system around 6,000 years ago among the ancient sages of India, and continues to be prized throughout the world today for the health benefits, happiness and mental serenity it brings.

Philosophy and meditation are intrinsic to the full practice of yoga, but here we are considering it for the opportunities it creates for full stretch workouts for the body's muscular core.

Simple yoga consists of a number of stances called asanas – positions named after an animal or, perhaps, human activity our bodies resemble when taking them up. Examples include the cat, dog, cobra, locust, corpse, tree, plough and warrior. You carry out the movements slowly and calmly, noting your breathing, and hold a posture only for as long as you comfortably can. Above all, you must avoid haste, tension, force and strain, all of which go against the principles of yoga. Yoga appeals to many couch potatoes because the more elementary asanas are easy to carry out and can be done almost anywhere, taking up very few minutes of your time.

You can go to a class or learn on your own or with a friend using a video, book or tape.

The asanas are great stress relievers, they're slow and peaceful and entirely non-competitive. Each of us practises yoga simply to the best of our ability, which makes it suitable for fit and unfit, young and old. By its very nature, yoga is carried out slightly differently by each of us because of our individual abilities and fitness levels, rather like the personal parameters of aerobic exercise, as discussed in Chapter 1. Things you find easy others will find hard and vice versa.

I shall now describe some easy yoga asanas and the benefits you can expect from them. Start by doing one or two, once a day, twice a week. Whenever you have time, start with the toning up technique which isn't exactly as you would do it in a yoga class, but sets the scene and mood for you, particularly on first waking. When you are familiar with these, slipping into them comfortably, add another, but note the following important consideration:

- If you suffer from any spinal or large joint problems, high blood pressure, heart disease or other serious or ongoing health problems, make certain to check first with your doctor or physiotherapist before trying any of the following.

Toning up

Sit comfortably on a carpeted floor or use a mat or rug. Using both hands, massage your scalp with your fingertips, then softly sweep your fingertips across the skin of your face and down the front of your throat. Gently massage the back of your neck and ears, the tops of your shoulders and shoulder blades as far back and down as you can reach, moving on to the very top of your chest on each side, just below the collar bones. Each time you complete an area, make gentle, sweeping, downward movements with your fingertips and the palms of your hands, towards the centre of your chest and upper abdomen over the solar plexus. Imagine you are drawing energy from all over your upper body into these areas, which are also the sites of two of the body's chakras, or energy centres, according to Indian philosophy.

Then turn your attention to the soles of both your feet and repeat the action, working up your body until you have covered every area, always sweeping invisible energy from each body part into the centre as before. You may be familiar with the technique of dry skin brushing, which many people do nowadays on a daily basis before showering, using a long-handled natural bristle body brush or loofah mitten. The purpose of dry skin brushing is to stimulate the skin and lymphatic system, speeding up the loss of toxic wastes through the skin, and improving the circulation and drainage of the lymphatic system.

The chief benefits of this toning up technique are the healthy stimulation of every bodily area and the increased release into the bloodstream of cancer-combating chemicals believed to accumulate over the body's surface throughout a night's sleep. Undoubtedly it provides the benefits of dry skin brushing as well.

Corpse position

Some people find this simple but important asana the most challenging of all because it demands physical stillness rather than action. Living in a busy, noisy and stressful world can render repose and silence almost intolerable to us when we first explore them. It is this obstacle that we have to overcome if we are to benefit fully from effortless exercise, because the activity and action must be counterbalanced by their opposite – relaxed joints and floppy, loose, slack muscles out of which all knots of irritation and anxiety readily flow. Take this medicine for five minutes, twice daily! Also do it before and after any exercising – relaxed muscles are less liable to be strained during exercise and enable it to be more beneficial. Relaxing after exercising helps you to unwind and provides a pause before you get on with the rest of your day.

Lie down on your back on a folded blanket or mat, with your arms a little way away from your body, palms upturned, and your heels slightly apart, feet turned gently out. Your spine should be straight, but keep a gentle curve at your waist – your back should not be arched or flat – and your hips should be level. Breathe slowly and deeply, allowing a feeling of calmness and ease to reach every part of your body. Concentrate on any areas of tension you may discover – typically in the abdomen, chest, shoulders, neck, facial muscles and tongue – and breathe them away as you breathe out. Follow these simple steps to help induce the relaxation you are seeking.

- Slowly inhale through your nostrils and, holding your breath, tense the muscles of your feet and toes. Breathe out, relaxing the tightened muscles as you do so.
- Slowly inhale and contract the muscles of your calves and knees,

as well as those of your feet and toes. Hold for a few seconds and tighten, really feeling the muscles pull. Breathe out and relax, experiencing fully the contrast between contraction and relaxation.

- Slowly inhale again, contracting your buttocks, pelvic muscles, hips and thighs, in addition to those of your calves, feet and toes. Relax and breathe out, again noting the contrast between muscular tightness and relaxation.

- Next, inhale, meanwhile tightening the muscles of your hand and fingers, wrists, elbows, lower and upper arms, shoulders and neck – as with the lower limbs, working inwards from the periphery (hands, wrists and so on) towards the centre of your body. Feel and identify the tightness of the contracted muscles in all the areas. Breathe out slowly and relax.

- Finally, inhale and contract the muscles of your scalp, and small muscles all over your face, including your ears, forehead, cheeks, chin and mouth. Wrinkle your nose, screw up your eyes tightly for a few seconds, clench your teeth, tighten the muscles of your throat, then stick out your tongue as far as you can without hurting its root. Hold and tighten your whole body, noting the almost intolerable tension. Exhale and relax. Relax fully and utterly. Notice how heavy and inert your body feels. Allow all the strain you have just surrendered to flow out of you into the floor. Above all, enjoy the relaxed muscle tone, the sensation of a boosted blood circulation and the new emotional calm.

In addition to learning how to relax (a much underrated life-saving skill!), reported benefits include improved circulation throughout the body to all its muscles and organs and the relief of fatigue, general exhaustion, nervousness and related anxiety disorders such as panic attacks. Others are the relief of asthma, constipation, indigestion, irritable bowel syndrome, lumbago and sleeping problems. Mental benefits include improved alertness and concentration, and greater emotional calm in the face of life's stresses and strains.

Kelly
Kelly is 45.

'I shall always be thankful to my yoga teacher for the many health benefits this stretching routine has given me over the years – especially in the first three months. Following a fall from my horse at a show, I was placed in traction for over a month and suffered from bad backaches and weak postural muscles when I came out of hospital. The osteopath I went to see once I was home strongly advised me to strengthen what he called my core muscles – those of the back and trunk. Yoga, she advised, was one of the best ways of achieving this.

'I was dubious about yoga's usefulness at first, having always been far more physically active than I feel this stretch exercise implies, but Marie, who took the yoga class, made sure we all had our individual requirements catered for in the asanas she taught the class. She would ask each of us to concentrate on certain positions and sit others out, as appropriate.

'The corpse appealed to me, because of its bizarre name and because it is extremely easy to do. Gradually I added other positions and remember that the locust and the cobra were especially useful for my weak and aching lower and upper back. In fact, the sensation of extending my spine while doing the cobra was just sensational after being immobilized for weeks in bed. I do a little routine of my own, including these three asanas, every day and still attend Marie's classes weekly.'

Knee roll

Lie down flat on your back with your arms by your sides. Gently raise your knees until they are touching the front of your chest or as close as you can get. Place your hands lightly on or around your knees. If you are too stiff, or carrying too much weight around your middle to be able to do this *do not fret and do not quit*! Get as close to this position as you can. You will soon make progress. Next, roll gently over on to your right side, move the arm you are now lying on out to the side to make yourself more comfortable and, keeping your legs and the side of your pelvis in stationary contact with the floor, twist your torso at the level of your waist and reach your upper left arm out to the left so that you are at least partly facing towards the left.

Turn as far as you comfortably can (some experts are flexible enough to get the left side of their head and face flat on the floor!) Hold this position for five to seven seconds (counting one thousand, two thousand and so on), then turn, again gently, until all your body is facing the same way, and return to your original lying down flat position. Rest for a few seconds, then repeat the actions on the left side. Build up to a total of five exercises each way in your own good time.

This exercises your chest, pelvic and upper and lower back muscles, as well as those of your thighs, neck and shoulders. Twisting the spine and main supporting trunk muscles at waist level improves flexibility, stamina and muscular strength.

Seat

A dull name for a simple manoeuvre that looks impressive once you've got the hang of it. Kneel upright then sit back on your heels, clasping your hands loosely in front of you in your lap. Then, without holding on to anything, keeping your back straight, and your knees on the floor, bring your upper body up slowly to an upright kneeling position – feel the muscles working through your thighs and contract your abdominal muscles to protect your back – hold this position for three seconds, then lower yourself slowly back down on to your heels once more. Do this twice. The aim is to strengthen your lower back, abdominal, thigh and torso muscles, making them sleeker and more efficient. The exercise should be performed smoothly, slowly and without pushing or jerking your shoulders forward or sticking your bottom out, in order to rise to an erect position. If this is impossible, hold on lightly to a piece of furniture that will stay put – not to pull yourself up, but to guide yourself through this movement.

Dave

Dave is 28.

'I was downgraded while in the RAF for three months following a viral illness. This meant that less was expected of me in terms of physical fitness and performance, but it also confined me to an office job after being active for years as a flight technician. I was sitting on an office stool in front of a computer for over 40 hours a week, and soon started to develop pains in my lower back and even sagging stomach muscles.

'The MO referred me to the camp physiotherapist, Peter, who gave me some simple strengthening exercises to do, based on yoga asanas. I had seen my sister doing them at home and thought yoga was for women – I was wrong! Two of the asanas were called the seat and the knee roll. Both were quite hard for me at first, because the virus had weakened and inflamed my muscles and because I had been sitting very badly at my office desk, in an effort to relieve my lower back pain.

'I had plenty of time to practise these two positions, and also the corpse (see above) – Peter stressed I must do them calmly and gently without straining, and also helped me correct my poor posture. After two to three weeks, my backache started to improve, and by the time I was upgraded once more and returned to my normal duties, my abdominal six-pack had returned. I still do the asanas several times a week, however. I find them great for destressing and helping me to relax.'

Cobra

This one makes you feel good straight away! Lie down on your front with your toes extended behind you. Place your hands, palms down, under your shoulders on the floor and keep your elbows tucked in. Then, while breathing in, but without raising your navel from the floor, lift your chest and head, *gently*, arching your back backwards until you just *start* to feel a pull in the muscles around your lower back – you should not feel any pinching or other pain. Keep your shoulders down, elbows in and your chin level, looking forwards. Retain your breath for five seconds, then exhale slowly while lowering yourself to the floor. Do this two or three times in all. Performed slowly and carefully, only going back as far as feels comfortable, you can feel the zipppp! of a boosted oxygen circulation and improved spinal flexibility almost immediately. Other reported benefits include relief for irregular periods and constipation, strengthened spinal muscles and a general toning effect.

Locust

First, it is important to note that you should avoid the locust position altogether if you have an acutely sore back or any kind of inflammatory disorder of the abdominal or pelvic organs, at least during flare-ups. However, the reputed benefits, other than muscle and joint flexibility and strengthening, are generally to the large and small bowel, so try it when you are feeling better and your doctor gives you the OK.

This is another easy asana to do, although hard to complete in full, at least initially. So don't try – just do what feels comfortable and you will soon make progress. Lie face down with your chin on the floor, clench your fists and move your arms and knuckles under you, pressing the floor down below your groin area so that you are supporting and partly lifting your pelvis. Breathe in, then, using your lower back muscles, raise one leg a little way towards the ceiling –

you shouldn't feel any pinching or pain in the back. Hold this for five to seven seconds, then exhale and relax, bringing the elevated leg back gently into position. Repeat this with the other leg. Do this one to three times – whatever you feel comfortable with. The more advanced form of the locust gets you raising both your legs at the same time – a strenuous undertaking and not to be attempted until you are generally more flexible and can raise each leg, locust-style, without stress or strain.

Pilates

Pronounced 'pee-la-tees', this exercise system was developed more than 60 years ago by the physical therapy innovator, Joseph Pilates (1880–1967). The co-ordinated movements tone and balance the muscles and help to realign displaced spinal and other joints. Like similar stretch routines, Pilates tones the core muscles of the torso and limbs, face and neck, as well as stimulating the central nervous system, the spinal nerves and the circulation. In fact, all Pilates activity is based on the eight principles of relaxation, concentration, alignment and breathing, co-ordination, centring, flowing movement and stamina, which, acting together, help to condition the body and mind, fight stress and decrease risks of injury.

Pilates is a popular health and beauty regimen, especially with people who have become disillusioned with the gym scene or who, like couch potatoes, have no wish to become acquainted with it. Its gentle, therapeutic approach makes it especially suitable for anyone recovering from an injury or debilitating illness. Its enthusiasts include many elderly people and others who haven't exercised for years, sportsmen and women wanting to reduce injury risks and/or improve their performance and anyone else with a need to stretch muscle groups that may escape attention during ordinary workouts. Pilates is also taught in some forward-looking mental health units where self-expression and stress reduction are especially important. In addition, many of its advocates claim that it has revolutionized their sex lives as a result of the muscle strengthening and toning, an increase in self-esteem and poise, and improved body outline and stamina they have experienced.

Pilates is also an excellent choice if you suffer from backache (but still check with a doctor or therapist first to make sure it's right in your personal circumstances) because it realigns and lengthens, strengthens and balances the spinal column and attached muscles. It can also help you if you're recovering from an operation or giving birth or suffer from arthritis in your main weight-bearing and similar joints, such as the hip, knee and shoulder.

You can learn Pilates from a class or video plus instruction book at home – sharing the experience may be most fun and more productive. Like yoga asanas, you only follow Pilates to top up your own personal strengths and improve the way you use your body in sports, when relaxing and at work, working only within your own capacity and fitness level. The core conditioning effect of Pilates (explained above) that develops the strength of the trunk is, in fact, based on the idea that, as a tree needs a strong trunk to survive the hazards of rough weather, so humans need a strong trunk to help them withstand physical and emotional stresses and carry out the thousand and one tasks we do daily, as efficiently as possible.

Rather than working on individual groups of muscles in isolation, Pilates tones, strengthens, improves posture and provides balance, flexibility and sound movement by working on the controlled movement of the spine and correct breathing. The main muscle groups targeted include the belt encircling the lower body, termed in Pilates 'the Powerhouse' – that is, those of the abdominal wall, lower back, hips and buttocks. You learn to contract, or squeeze, the muscles in turn, for optimal core strength and stability (thereby avoiding a shortcoming found in some other core programmes where an inappropriate sequence of squeezes can leave the spine as unstable as it was before).

The advantages of improved core strength soon become apparent, enabling the correctly functioning posture muscles to work more efficiently, doing less work and utilizing less oxygen and energy in the process.

Here are some examples of the sequences you can try. Wear comfortable clothing that allows free movement, remain barefoot or wear socks and use a padded mat. A long scarf, a firm, flat pillow or folded towel and a tennis ball may be required for some of the exercises.

Checking your alignment

It is important to do this first. When your body is in alignment:

- your pelvis is in neutral – tipped neither forwards nor backwards;
- your spine is lengthened, but still with its natural curves;

- shoulders are down – the shoulder-blades slid down into your back;
- neck is released and soft, the back of the neck staying long;
- feet are hip-width apart and parallel.

Breathing

In Pilates, you breathe into your lower ribcage and back, feeling your back widening, so as to maximize lung capacity. This increases your oxygen intake, creates greater flexibility in your upper body and works on your abdominal area.

This is how to do it. Sit, stand or kneel in alignment, wrap the scarf around your ribcage, cross the ends over in front and pull gently to feel where you are working. The idea is to breathe into your scarf, directing your breath into your sides and back rather than letting your upper chest expand as it normally does. Feel the ribs go in and out and use your abdominal muscles too, as you exhale and inhale. Relax and breathe softly, six times in all.

Creating a strong centre

To strengthen and stabilize your core muscles, get on to your hands and knees, your knees under your hips, your hands under your shoulders, looking down or slightly in front of you, still looking at the floor. Breathe into your back as described above to prepare and lengthen throughout the spine. Breathe out and squeeze the muscles of your abdomen and pelvic floor (as described on page 35), pulling your lower abdominal muscles back towards your lower spine. Breathe in again and relax. This is similar to the feeling when you are zipping up a close-fitting pair of jeans, keeping your pelvic and tummy organs in position.

Morning stretch and relaxation position

Sit on the floor as though you were going to sit cross-legged but instead put the soles of your feet together (or as close to each other as you comfortably can). You can make sure your pelvis is correctly positioned by sitting with your lower back against a wall. Breathe in, then out, as before, pulling up your imaginary zip and pulling in your belly button, while relaxing forward. Hinge forwards from your hips, keeping your back straight, in alignment, not hunched over as this puts strain on your back. Only go as far forward as you can without straining while still maintaining alignment, bringing your chest towards your knees. Take ten breaths into your lower ribcage and back in this folded position, keeping your neck lengthened and arms resting in front of you without humping your shoulders.

Then, with your abdominal muscles contracted as before to protect your back, slowly unfurl as you breathe out, fully lengthening your spine and keeping it in alignment.

A tip for feeling great in the morning is to try this stretch on getting out of bed, after you have stretched all over as explained in the previous chapter before getting out of bed.

The starfish

Lie on your back with your knees bent, feet a hip width apart, soles flat on the floor and with your arms by your sides. Place a small flat pillow or folded towel under your head if you want to ensure that your face is parallel with the floor. Breathe in and out as described earlier and feel yourself widening and lengthening. Breathe in to prepare, then out using the zip technique, keeping your back in neutral, and, while exhaling, slide your right leg away from you straight ahead along the floor, at the same time taking your left arm back, gently, so that it touches the floor behind you, if you comfortably can. Stretch gently forward and back as if someone were pulling your outstretched feet away from each other.

Repeat five times a side, always ensuring that you do not hump your shoulders, your neck remains relaxed and your pelvis stays in neutral.

As this releases tension and misalignment throughout your spine and lower back, you might like to do the starfish when you get in from work in the evening or after a long day at home busy with children and housework. Also try having a warm bath or shower beforehand as this loosens the muscles, enabling you to derive maximum benefit from this stretch exercise.

Shoulder drop

Lie on your back in the relaxation position described at the beginning of the starfish exercise above and breathing into the back as before. Raise both arms towards the ceiling directly above your shoulders and with their palms facing each other. Imagine you are trying to reach for the ceiling with one arm – stretching right up your arm into your fingertips. Once your shoulder blade has left the floor, return your arm to the relaxation position. Repeat ten times for each arm: this is great for easing shoulder and neck tension.

You can increase the tension-easing effect by inhaling some

essential oil of lavender. To pep you up and increase mental alertness afterwards, try inhaling a little essential oil of peppermint, rosemary or basil on a tissue tucked into your jacket pocket or bra.

Liz
Liz is 55.

'I have always suffered from a stiff neck and upper back – partly because, at 5 foot 11, I am very tall for a woman and became used, early in life, to hunching my shoulders to avoid sticking out like a sore thumb.

'When I started working from home as a proof-reader after my son was born, the pain in my shoulders and neck nearly drove me mad. I realized I was not sitting as I should at the computer, but even when I tried to improve my sitting posture, nothing improved.

'Then a girlfriend asked me to join her in learning some Pilates from a videotape she had been given – it had a book with it, so that we could read as well as look and listen. I soon learned how much benefit could be gained from simple exercises such as the starfish, shoulder drops and the morning stretch. It hurt at first even to attempt them, but my doctor checked my spine and told me I should persist.

'Now I practise a 15-minute routine every morning without fail, before the rest of the house wakes. I wouldn't be without Pilates for the world and, best of all, the positions are about gentle stretching and relaxation; they do not demand any effort.'

Anthony
Anthony is 75.

'You may not think an old chap like me would be enthusiastic about exercise, nor have time for new fangled stretches and the like, but my granddaughter, aged 18, started this thing called Pilates and was telling me about it when my back was very sore. I had also recently developed an inguinal hernia in my right groin.

'She told me that Pilates was for people of all ages and that she thought it could benefit me. She said it strengthened the muscles of the abdominal wall and lower back – and my doctor had told me my hernia was partly due to weak tummy muscles. Well, I did as she showed me, very gently – in fact, we did "my" exercises for twenty minutes a time, three times a week for the first month. Nothing hurt or felt over-stretched and I really enjoyed myself. I felt younger and livelier, and my back was less troublesome.

'It was also a huge bonus when my doctor examined me three months after I had started Pilates and told me that my abdominal wall had strengthened sufficiently for me not to need surgery for my hernia. So I have several good reasons to be grateful to my granddaughter and to Pilates stretch exercise.'

5

Working *With* Resistance

Hopefully, by now, most couch potato readers are coming round to the view that a little, regular, *gentle* exercise might be worth including in their lives, considering its life-saving benefits, anti-ageing effects, fat-busting qualities, figure-honing actions and depression-beating reputation, of course! So, here we shall look at different sorts of resistance exercise and decide whether or not – and, if so, how – to include it in our scheme.

As you may know, resistance exercise, also known as weight training, is the sort of thing people get up to in gyms, such as when they are circuit training (going around a circuit of weighted machines – see below – and exercising for a specified time on each in turn). An image may therefore spring to mind, in association with resistance work, of a huge, sweaty man or woman with sculpted biceps and pectoral muscles (*pecs*, as they call them), struggling and grunting as they heave at massive metal dumb-bells. I must dispel this picture from your mind right away!

As you have never contemplated visiting a gym – and there is absolutely no need to do so, I promise – you may wonder why I bother to include such a picture here. Trust me! I simply want to give you an idea of what takes place in gyms and such places so that you can compare it with the far gentler resistance ideas I will give you for use at home, at work or wherever you happen to be when you have a few minutes to spare.

One glimpse inside a busy gym, in fact, on a weekday evening is enough to put most timid souls off their supper and ensure that the only time they exercise aerobically thereafter is when jogging smartly past the gym's front door! The last thing I am going to do is scare you by launching into an impassioned support of heavy breathers wherever they happen to congregate. Before you label this patronizing, please let me repeat again and again that there really is no *need* to wave metal weights around in the air or submit yourself to apparatus that looks as though it has come from a torture chamber just to gain the benefits of resistance. They are all yours for the taking and you can obtain them without coming anywhere close to weight-laden iron bars. Without, in fact, even noticing that you're exercising at all.

I should also mention that you will not develop those massive muscles of which bodybuilders are so proud (see below). All most of us are really after is improved health and fitness, plus a leaner, flab-free outline and much more energy. Without making any effort. Right then . . .

What is resistance work?

Resistance exercise is so called because it makes us work against some type of self-imposed, self-regulated force that offers some resistance. This can be as challenging or as easy as we choose. As I mentioned earlier, within the gym environment, weighted machines provide most of the resistance and it is usual to set these at a certain level so that the muscles are working against so many pounds or kilograms of weight. The kind of resistance activity we will be doing here, though, is more casual, consisting of, for instance, pressing against and away from a wall or, very frequently, the force of gravity – when doing sit-ups, for instance, bridging or Superman (see below). The resistance gravity provides is especially useful because the amount of effort we have to make to combat it, such as repetitions of leg-raises, is automatically in proportion to our level of fitness, the weight of the limb concerned, and the number of repetitions we attempt in any one stint.

The benefits of resistance

Like the other types of exercise we have looked at, resistance training has the potential to build, strengthen and tone muscles, as well as increase stamina. It is especially good, when used correctly, at shaping and toning muscles to produce a sleeker outline. Resistance work also develops lean body mass (which is especially important if you are trying to lose weight, because it uses up more food energy as fuel than does fatty tissue, which in turn promotes the burning of stored fat layers and weight loss), increases co-ordination and balance, helps to strengthen bones against osteoporosis (brittle bone disease) and reduces the risks of injury from muscular weakness. Whether you become bulkier as a result of resistance training or just more flexible and toned depends on your sex, age, hormone levels and, of course, how much and how strenuously you exercise.

Just to reassure you – although this is, of course, likely to be academic for readers of this book – the male hormone testosterone encourages muscles to increase in size and bulk, which is what men tend to experience with regular weight training, but male readers doing the resistance exercises described below will only become more toned without that bodybuilder look. Women, who also secrete testosterone but in much smaller quantities, will tend to become firmer, stronger and more slender (especially where excess body fat has been shed), but not excessively so. You can rest assured that you will not end up looking muscle-bound just because you include some resistance activity in your schedule – assuming, I am sure safely, that you stay off anabolic steroids and don't follow a fanatical exercise regime.

A gym of your own?

Perhaps you have imagined having your own private gym, maybe with an attractive personal trainer thrown in, but banished the dream to a fantasy world in which you also win the lottery? Although not as sleek, our homespun, but nevertheless very effective, types of resistance activity mean you can, if you wish, create a pretty good gym in your own home, with a little imagination and ingenuity. Find somewhere you can work out in peace, without feeling self-conscious about being a raw beginner and or having to fork out loads of money for fashionable gear. You could do your exercises before everyone else wakes up, while lunch is cooking or while the children are at school. As for the attractive instructor, well, you can either work with your partner, giving your mutual erotic fantasies a new lease of life, or give yourself a makeover when your body looks the way you want it before searching once more for a mate.

If you aren't looking, that's fine! You will only stick with effortless (or any other sort of) exercise long enough to make any difference if you are doing it primarily for *yourself*. You, after all, are the worthiest cause of all.

Incidentally, planning a complete makeover or other special treat for when you see and feel great results is an excellent spur to continuing with your plan. However, there is no need whatsoever to wait – try giving yourself little treats along the way. These provide excellent boosts to morale and determination and also help pick you up if you have meandered off the path of your good intentions. I will be giving you ideas for interim rewards and bonus tips throughout this chapter.

Home props

Here are some ways in which the normal, everyday features of any home (or office) can provide useful resistance for you to work with.

- *Walls* can be used to test and maintain posture (providing they are straight to start off with!).
- *Sofas, tables and chairs* are useful 'steadiers' for practising squats and other weight-related exercises.
- *Food and drinks tins* make excellent hand weights. Start with slim, lighter tins of, for instance, tonic water or fruit juice, to get used to handling these while exercising. Progress to fatter, heavier tins when you are ready.
- *The bottom stair* makes a great platform for step exercises. If you live in a bungalow, try piling several telephone directories on top of one another to a height of about 15 cm (6 in). Alternatively, use a safe (non-fragile) wooden box, and make sure it won't slide when you step up and down on it.
- *Home exercise equipment* can be bought once you feel committed enough to know that you will use it. Advertisements for many different types abound in newspapers and magazines, on TV and so on, but I suggest that you first try my ideas, any of which you can put into practice with little or no preparation, whenever you feel like it and without spending any money or very little.

Exercising with resistance

Quarter squats

Here is an exercise for whenever and wherever to strengthen thigh, lower back and abdominal muscles.

Stand with your feet about hip-width apart and dip down gently so that you are in a semi (or actually quarter) squatting position. Rest your hands on a chair back or other piece of *stable* furniture to steady yourself if you like, but don't hang on so tightly that you don't feel your legs are doing any work. Pretend that you are going to squat right down on your heels but, instead, only slightly flex your thigh muscles so that you are partially squatting.

Hold the position for a count of two seconds (say to yourself, one thousand, two thousand), then slowly and gently straighten up. Keep your back as straight as you can and avoid leaning forwards or backwards, and your pelvis in neutral. Imagine you are lowering yourself on to a seat below your bottom. Then, pushing yourself up with your thighs, and your bottom muscles, straighten up. Repeat – five times altogether.

One steps

This exercise also strengthens the thigh and calf muscles, lower abdomen and lower back.

Organize your step prop – the bottom step of a staircase or books piled up safely as suggested above and so on. Step up using your right foot, pause for a second as your left foot joins it. Then step down again with the right foot and down again to the floor with your left. Do this ten times, say, then do another set of repetitions (the same number), starting with your left foot.

Reward yourself

When you have done your quarter squats and one steps daily for a week, reward yourself with a home pedicure. Soak in a warm bath, towel yourself dry then, sitting comfortably in a good light, clip or file your toenails, push back the cuticles using cuticle cream if necessary, rub in some moisturizer and coat each nail with your favourite or a new nail polish. For men, instead of varnish, buff your toenails with a purpose-made chamois buffer for a natural and healthy shine.

Bonus tip

Do you have sore, aching feet? Feel exhausted and under the weather? Suffer from arthritis, migraine, PMS, period problems or other disorders that plague you? Make an appointment with a qualified reflexologist (check in your local *Yellow Pages* or ask around to get a personal recommendation). Not only will your feet receive a thorough working over, but low energy levels and long-term chronic conditions may also improve too. Reflexologists examine and massage the feet to locate and free blocked energy pathways from all areas and organs of the body that can be held by complementary therapists to cause illness.

Repeat these two rewards every few weeks, for happier feet and overall health.

Anna

Anna is 28.

'I had been inactive for about ten years, when I started to get pains in my lower back and legs. I went to my doctor and he said I probably wasn't exercising enough – I played in the hockey first eleven at school – and advised me to go jogging.

'This was very bad news because I did what he said and simply ended up with worse pain and stiffness than before.

'Then my father, who had had a road traffic accident and spent months in bed, suggested I see his physiotherapist. She – Suzanne – told me I was in no fit state to jog or run and advised me to do resistance exercises to strengthen my muscles and regain my former fitness. One thing she taught me I shall always remember – that was to challenge first the main muscles that contribute to movement. She advised lots of quarter squats, and also daily step exercises using a couple of telephone directories.

'This didn't seem to do anything for me at first, but I soon noticed the benefit when I persisted, and I could actually feel my thigh and lower leg, lower tummy and lower back muscles regaining their old strength. As I went on with these, Suzanne taught me other resistance exercises to do and soon I was back to the old form I was in while at school. I do these and other resistance exercises every day now and have also taken up simple aerobic exercise once more to help return me to my old, fit self. Combined with yoga, I have to say that resistance work – however simple – got me going again and nowadays I wouldn't be without it.'

Sit-ups

Let's face it, we all would like flat or flatter stomachs. There are several resistance exercises that can have this effect and, even though they don't require much effort, they will produce results. The one rule is that you have to do them regularly over a period of months – and then keep them up! Try sit-ups and Superman below and see for yourself.

Lie on your back on a firm, flat surface – on a towel, or rug, on the floor is ideal. Bend your knees up and put your feet flat on the floor. Then, prepare as described for the Pilates exercises earlier in this chapter, breathing and contracting your abdomen, and slide your hands up your thighs gradually and slowly, raising your head, neck and upper torso as you do so, curling in towards your chest. Raise yourself *only* as far as you comfortably can, hold for a second or two, then s-l-o-w-l-y lower yourself down again to your starting position. Repeat five times. It is important to pull your tummy in towards your back rather than let it dome – if it does this, do not travel so far up your legs until your muscles are stronger. Also, you should not feel any pain in your back – again, do not aim to lift so high if this happens. If you do this exercise regularly, you'll be surprised at how quickly your muscles become more toned.

Superman!

Lie on your tummy and raise and stretch out first your right arm and your left leg – only as far as you comfortably can and certainly lower them a little if there is any pinching or pain in your back. Breathe and contract your abdominal muscles as described for the Pilates exercises and hold for two to three seconds (counting one thousand, two thousand, and so on). Repeat, using your left arm and right leg. Do a total of five per side.

This feels odd at first, as though you are using a huge amount of effort and not shifting at all. Untrue! This exercise stretches your abdominal, buttock and thigh muscles, making them work and letting you feel them pulling against gravity as you go into the movement. If you enjoy this – and I think you will – repeat at least once daily and start to notice the benefits in your improved tummy outline.

Reward yourself

You're now adding repetitions of sit-ups and the Superman exercise too the quarter squats and one steps above. When you are doing all four types as a matter of course, four to six days a week, reward yourself – you're doing brilliantly, you deserve it!

Buy yourself some gorgeous underwear – lingerie, boxer shorts, whatever feels special – choose the best you can afford! You will doubtless buy more in the months to come, to celebrate your toned lower half, but now is the time to give yourself a taste of future glory! Don't just keep these delightful garments in a drawer for 'best'; you want to feel and look your best every day (you're already making great progress in this direction!) – so put them on and feel wonderful *now*!

Bonus tip

Wage war on any cellulite on your thighs, tummy or buttocks. Buy a product based on natural ingredients, such as ivy extract, mud or seaweed. Use according to the instructions, remembering to stroke or brush your abdomen *gently* in a clockwise direction if you include this area in your treatment.

Include foods that specifically burn fat in your daily diet for two weeks, to boost the loss of stored fat layers naturally. Examples include first-class protein cooked without fat – lean meat and poultry, fish, eggs, cottage cheese and soya products, such as tofu – and low GI (glycaemic index) foods that raise the body's glucose and energy levels slowly – sweet potatoes, okra, broccoli, brown rice, wild rice, pearl barley, multigrain (brown or white) bread, heavy fruit breads, bananas, apples and grapefruit, for example.

Bob

Bob is 40.

'I really lost my nice, neat figure after I stopped playing football and taking advantage of the many exercises our manager gave us to do. This was when I was 27 and decided that I hadn't really got what it takes to be a premier league player. The trouble was, I gave up exercise in a huff and really let myself go. I put on 2 stone (13 kg) in weight, and my weakened stomach muscles made me look as though I was nine months pregnant.

'Then I met the girl I wanted to marry. Chrissy was on top form, being a personal trainer and having about a dozen men and women waiting on her every word to improve their fitness and stamina. I didn't think I stood a chance with her, but she clearly saw something in me, because she came over one evening when I was doing some rather futile press-ups in the park and asked me why I was exercising in such a negative way! I had seen her at the gym, but had never actually spoken to her.

'What she told me not only revitalized my fitness programme, but also helped us to get together. She advised me not to do stupid press-ups all on my own, but to exercise intelligently, including less stressful types of resistance or weight training in my plan. I did what she suggested, including stomach-strengthening exercises, to get me back to my old form.

'Superman lifts and sit-ups were only part of it. These strengthened my tummy muscles and helped restore their six-pack look. I had nothing to lose, beyond about 10 surplus pounds of fat (4.5 kg), so I put myself in Chrissy's capable hands. When I had finished my course with her, I asked her out and she said 'yes' at once. We have been together for ten years now – a day does not pass without our exercising together and I can honestly say that agreeing to do abdominal strengthening exercises paved the way to our happiness today.'

Bridging

This and the following are brilliant exercises for toning and firming your bottom and the backs of your thighs, your hamstrings. They strengthen them too, making activities such as climbing stairs, hill walking and cycling less of a bind.

Lie down flat on the floor on your back, on a rug or soft mat. With a chair in front of your feet, leave one leg where it is on the floor and rest the heel of the other on the edge of the seat of the chair, keeping that leg straight.

Raise the 'floor' leg and foot as high as you comfortably can, keeping your bottom on the floor, five times. Change legs and repeat the raising exercise on the other side. This stretches and works the gluteus maximus muscles of the buttocks and the hamstrings of the raising leg.

Side-steps

This makes further use of your improvised step apparatus (the bottom stair, small platform, stable pile of telephone directories or whatever else you've chosen).

Stand sideways on your step, with one foot on the floor. Step up on to it five times, then turn round and repeat with the other leg. Do this four to five times in all to start with, slowly increasing the number as you feel comfortable.

Reward yourself

Your favourite upbeat music playing while you do this will boost your energy levels and cheer you on as you're exercising. This applies, of course, to any of the aerobic or resistance exercises we have looked at, but you might like to try it out for the first time when using your step 'machine'. Outside the home, you can do this exercise wherever you find a spare stair, but avoid public staircases when in use by other people!

You can use music to excellent advantage after exercising as well. Have a long soak in lovely, warm, scented water (add a few drops of ylang ylang essential oil for a wonderful aroma and sense of peace, or burn a scented candle – rose, clove and other spices, sandalwood, vanilla and freesia are all excellent). Finally, choose gentle, soothing music to suit this scene and that uplifts your spirits.

Bonus tip

Pour yourself something tasty to sip, pleasuring all five senses as you soak. Note the delicious contrast between your chilled drink and the warm, steamy atmosphere!

Lime sparkler

Chill 300 ml (½ pint) tumbler beforehand, if you remember. Carefully pare a long curl of peel from a very fresh lime (avoid all pith) and place it in the tumbler together with the squeezed juice of half of the fruit. Add several ice cubes, top with sparkling mineral water, add a good pinch of salt (which will make it foam) and stir vigorously. Sip as you lie back, congratulating yourself on your recent exercise. Any sparkling mineral water will do, but I find this works especially well with Perrier water.

Spicy perry

Chill a large wine glass in advance. Add a couple of ice cubes, three cloves with their heads bashed to release their oils, a cinnamon stick and a pinch of ground nutmeg. Pour over some chilled, sparkling perry, use the cinnamon stick to stir it all round, then discard. Sip, reflecting philosophically on the finer things in your life. Don't bother to try to fish out the cloves – you'll miss out on soaking time and you can always discard them if you get them in your mouth.

To spice things up even further, try burning a spice candle while you sip this drink – you can find gorgeous, chunky ones containing whole slices of orange, citrus peel, bay leaves, cinnamon and cloves. Alternatively, heat a few drops of a spicy essential oil mixture in an aromatherapy burner or simply add them to your bathwater.

Jane

Jane is 19 years old.

'I wasn't exactly overweight as a child – just stocky, I suppose you'd call it – but I started to get teased about my shape when I changed schools at the age of 13. I wasn't keen on games or PE and hated them even more when we had to change in front of one another in the cloakrooms. My thighs were shapeless and my bottom, I have to admit, did tend to stick out, and I was christened

"Thunder Thighs" and "Big Bum". In the end I loathed going to school so much that I started to play truant, but it wasn't until one of the mistresses saw me at the shops during school hours that anything was said.

'My parents were upset with me when they heard, but were even more upset when I told them why I was developing school phobia. I had some counselling, which was brilliant at boosting my self-esteem, and my mother – ever the pragmatist – said we would beat the bullies at their own game! All she meant by this was that she would get someone to show me exercises that would help reshape my ungainly figure, but her positive help and encouragement spurred me on to make the necessary effort.

'Our family doctor wasn't interested – he just said I would grow out of my big bottom and thighs and, if I didn't, I would have to learn to live with them. So Mum booked some private lessons with a personal trainer at her gym and she, Katy, showed me some good exercises to do. Side-steps and bridging were my favourites – I used to put the stereo on in my room or take a radio outside to the garage, close the doors and turn up the volume. I slowly built up my reps [repetitions] until I was exercising for 20 minutes or so 5 or 6 days a week.

'Results weren't immediate, but every week I would examine my hips, bottom and thighs, just wearing tights, in my full-length bedroom mirror and it wasn't all that long before I began to notice some difference. I also measured my hips and thighs before starting and then every month – I lost 2 in (5 cm) off each thigh and 3 in (7.5 cm) off my hips. I also shed half a stone (3 kg) in weight, although I had not set out to do this. The teasing dwindled away when I stopped reacting to the unkind comments and, a year on, one of the girls responsible actually came and asked me what exercises I had been doing – "I had such a neat rear and she wouldn't mind following suit!" Soon a whole load of us were exercising to firm and strengthen offending parts of our bodies and, two years after leaving school, we are all still friends.'

Wall push-ups

This and the remaining exercises in this chapter provide some resistance work for the upper half of your body.

Wall push-ups strengthen and tone the muscles of your shoulders, upper arms (biceps at the front and triceps at the back) and forearms.

Stand facing a wall, about 30 to 40 cm (12 to 15 in) away. Place both hands flat on the wall at about shoulder height and, keeping your feet still, lean forwards slowly keeping your body in a straight line and your shoulders down until your forehead is quite close to the wall. Hold for a second or two, then push back gently until you regain your original position. Start with five of these and build up to ten or however many you enjoy doing without overstraining. If you find this easy, stand a bit further away from the wall, gradually increasing the distance as you get stronger, but be careful not to lock your elbows; keep a bit of give in them to protect the joints.

Biceps curl

No exercise targets one muscle or group of muscles exclusively, but these curls are aimed at strengthening and toning the biceps – they stretch the triceps at the same time, of course.

Depending on your size and strength, choose small tonic water or fruit juice tins or larger, heavier tins of fruit or baked beans.

Stand well balanced and facing forwards, your feet about a shoulder-width apart. Holding a can in each hand in front of you at waist level, palms upwards, raise one up to shoulder height by bending your elbow. As you lower this hand, raise the other and so on. Do ten repetitions in all, slowly building up to whatever you feel comfortable with.

Reward yourself

If you have always disliked the shape of your upper arms and tend to avoid sleeveless tops even in the warmest weather, then you have a particular incentive to do these exercises. Start by measuring each upper arm – write the figure in your diary or a notebook – and repeat every month after exercising regularly. Reward yourself as soon as your arms become a tiny bit more shapely, perhaps buying an attractive top with loose-fitting sleeves shorter than you would normally choose – nothing too daring, but pleasant to wear. Then, as these and other exercises produce further effects, experiment with shorter and shorter sleeves until you find a new style you are comfortable with. Finally, when you think you have achieved all the results you're going to achieve, try a sleeveless top. To grow used to this, you could start with a new nightie or cheap, casual top to wear around the house. It will not be long before you feel confident enough about your new, improved shape to wear anything you want with panache and pleasure!

Bonus point

Remember to eat at least five portions of fruit and vegetables daily (preferably fresh). The antioxidant vitamins and minerals these supply help to fight cellulite by counteracting the effects of free radicals, which are one of the main causes of tissue damage, including that of the lymphatic vessels, which help to drain excess fluid and toxic waste substances away from areas such as the upper arms, buttocks and thighs. Fresh, raw vegetables and fruit also fight flabbiness by aiding the body to shed surplus fat and retained fluid. You can easily increase your intake of raw plant foods by basing one meal a day around a large, raw salad or by substituting for high-fat, high-sugar snacks raw baby carrots or alfalfa, or mung bean sprouts.

Audrey
Audrey is 68.

'I have bred and shown pug dogs all my life and have taught ring craft for the past 15 years. Consistent training, understanding your dogs and knowing how to present their best features – are all important to prize winning, but it helps if the dog handler has a neat, attractive outline as well! I always did until I was off the show scene for a year fighting ovarian cancer. Thank God – and the medical and nursing staff and my family – I pulled through, but being inactive for several months played havoc with my figure, especially the tops of my arms where a lot of flab gathered.

'Fat arms had never been one of my problems and I was aghast, and probably hypersensitive, too, at the way I looked. I was eating healthily and starting to exercise once more, but I hadn't enough energy – nor would my doctors have approved, if I had – to undertake strenuous resistance work at the gym. I was particularly upset because my muscles felt weak and wobbly as well, and I found the dogs' pulling, even quite gently, on their leads a strain on my upper and lower arms.

'My eldest daughter came to my rescue. She is a physiotherapist and lives in Australia, but came home for the summer when my cancer was diagnosed and remained with me long enough after I recovered to give me some good advice. She said "little and often" should be my motto and that a few reps each day of carefully chosen exercises would – if I were persistent and patient! – bring about the changes I felt desperate to see.

'Choosing two little cans of fruit juice, I started on daily bicep curls – ten reps a day each side, five or six days a week. When these started to feel light, I changed to cans of vegetables, fruit or juice – always something my husband and I enjoyed eating or drinking afterwards! In fact we made a really childish game of it – I would choose two tins of an appropriate size every Saturday at the supermarket and John would ask me during the week if I could just "toss up" a quick snack for him or "whizz up" something to drink! It's astonishing what two people in love (after forty years of marriage) will find to giggle at!

'We experimented with lots of things we hadn't tried before – bamboo shoots, water chestnuts, artichoke hearts, mango slices, lychees ... we included many of these in salads and actually started eating even more healthily as a result!

'Anyway, the biceps curls gradually strengthened my biceps and I could lead the dogs again, in and out of the show ring, as often as I chose without becoming fatigued. As for the wall press-ups, I got John doing them too and, although he didn't need to lose any fat from his upper arms, he said he thought they did him a lot of good! The two exercises, between them, I am delighted to say, helped to remould my flabby upper arms and I soon regained all my old confidence and flair for exhibiting and showing my darling pugs.'

Carver chair

This is especially good for the shoulders, upper arms and forearms.

Sit in a typical carver dining chair – that is, an upright chair with arms – with your feet flat on the floor in front of you and your hands on the arm rests. Gently raise yourself, lifting your bottom a little from the seat and letting your arms do the work in propelling you upwards. Hold for a few seconds, then gently lower yourself back to your sitting position.

Prayer mat

Kneel on the floor in front of a prayer or other mat (1 m by 46 cm/ $3\frac{1}{2}$ feet by 18 in) with its short side towards you (if you don't have one, don't worry – you can do the exercise on any rug or carpet). Sit on your heels, then go on to your hands and knees. With your hands on the floor underneath your shoulders, bend your arms at the elbows and lower your upper body down slowly, keeping your back straight, until your face is a little above the mat – it's a bit like doing a press-up. Hold for a couple of seconds and then raise yourself back up, pushing up with your arms and hands, until you are once more on your hands and knees, but do not lock your elbows, keep them soft. Do this five times to start with, gradually increasing the number until you are doing, say, ten or so per set of repetitions.

Reward yourself

Further congratulations are in order once you have included the last two resistance exercises in your regular programme and a further reward is also appropriate! As by this time you are probably doing some regular aerobic manoeuvres, some stretching and/or some resistance activity, all in the comfort and privacy of your home, why not splurge on some really delectable exercise kit that you will look forward to wearing daily (or however many times a week are appropriate). Having spent a little (though quite enough!) time in gyms to watch how others go about obtaining the benefits for which they pay so highly, I am convinced that, for some members at least, walking around in fancy gear, sipping bottled water with a towel round their necks is what actually turns them on. Well, you are a legitimate exerciser of the effortless type, so are even more entitled to a bit of designer glam. My advice is go for it and remind yourself, every time you feel like changing into your new clothes, what a long way you have come from being a couch potato.

Bonus tip

If you feel like treating yourself on the culinary front as well – and why not? – here are two very simple meals based on first-class protein with a minimum of saturated fat.

Fillet steak a-caper
Serves 1
100–175 g (4–6 oz) fillet steak, trimmed of any gristle and fat
1 teaspoon olive oil
handful of button mushrooms, wiped and sliced
1–2 vine tomatoes, sliced
sea salt and freshly ground black pepper to taste
1 tablespoon capers

Heat a (preferably non-stick) frying pan with a heavy base and a lid until its interior is far too hot to touch, then add the olive oil and, a second or two later, the fillet steak. Spear the meat with a fork and use it to spread the oil around the pan. Turn the steak over, add the mushrooms, tomatoes and all their juice and a grinding of sea salt and black pepper, cover and cook over medium heat for 4–5 minutes, until the vegetables have cooked in the steam. Remove the lid, stir the contents of the pan to mingle all the juices, toss in the capers, remove and serve on a hot plate with a simple watercress and fresh orange salad.

Even simpler plaice
Serves 1
1 large plaice fillet
2 heaped tablespoons cooked basmati rice
1 finely sliced garlic clove
1 teaspoon olive oil
1 medium courgette, sliced

Place fish on a microwave-safe plate, cover and cook in the microwave on medium heat for about 2 minutes (it is done when the translucent flesh has become opaque and flakes easily). Keep warm, while you heat the oil in a frying pan and cook the garlic over a medium heat, adding the courgette slices after a minute and stirring to avoid them burning. Add the rice to heat it, just as the vegetables are done, then tip on to a plate and eat with the plaice.

If you find the plaice a bit bland, add a few flakes of fresh ginger root or some Japanese light soy sauce.

Jake
Jake is 31.

'My arm and shoulder muscles started to get very tight when I took up an office job after leaving school. I sat crouched at my desk all day and rarely got up and stretched, although I knew I should. That was during my gap year, and when I got to university and wanted to take up table tennis again, I found I just did not have the stamina.

'I play to county standard and went to our coach in despair. He discovered that I had really become unfit while confined to the office atmosphere – I had no spur to keep at sports when all my friends were out of town – and gave me a customized remedial programme to get me back on form. I had to do some aerobic exercise, regular bending and stretching – including yoga – and some resistance work to help my shoulders, upper back and especially my upper arms, biceps and triceps.

'Prayer mat and carver chair were so good to do! I could feel the strength and tone returning to my weakened muscles, and I was able to return to competition table tennis at the beginning of my second term at university.'

6
Exercising Your Choices

To get the best out of exercising, you need to fit it into your working or leisure hours without fuss or strain. Hopefully, you will find the tips in this and previous chapters useful. You also need a healthy diet to provide masses of energy, sound sleep and a good chunk of 'personal time out' daily, for pleasure and to combat stress. Finally, I include the words of those who have experienced the positive effects that the exercises described in this book have had on their lives.

On waking

Very few of us enjoy getting up in the morning (or after our main sleep for those of us who work shifts). This is especially true of the night owls among us who come to life as the day draws in and dusk settles. Even larks, who are far brighter than sleepy owls on waking, have been known to pull the duvet over their heads when their alarm goes off on cold winter mornings.

It may, therefore, demand an effort of will to get up earlier than usual. Please believe me, though – this from someone who loathes mornings – that it truly is worthwhile. Aim at just 15 minutes earlier to start with and begin by wriggling down the bed as described in Sharon's case history (see pages 30–31). If you have a partner who is still asleep, at least you won't disturb them. If you sleep alone or your partner doesn't mind, switch on the light if it's still dark or a dull day. This tells your system that you mean business! You could also try placing your alarm clock or radio out of reach so that you have to get out of bed to switch it off.

Once on your feet and having already loosened up a little, you can put on the kettle and make a hot drink (see below). Do another couple of stretches while it cools – toning up, knee roll and/or seat (see pages 47, 50, 51, 56) are all good choices. However, I recommend that you avoid the corpse asana first thing if you have problems waking – it is so calming you will probably nod off again!

As you start your day

What are you normally doing at 8.15 a.m. on a weekday? Heading for the office, shop, factory, hospital, garden centre or wherever you work? Doing the school run? Starting on the housework? Wherever you are, organize a ten-minute brisk walk for yourself. Get off the bus or tube, or park the car, a couple of stops further from work or school (the children need the exercise as much as you).

If your time is your own, simply slip on a coat and start walking. Head round the block, across the park, down the lane or, if you are lucky enough to have a large garden or field, stride around that a few times instead. The exercise will pep up your energy levels, the fresh air will get your brain buzzing and Nature could well provide you with unexpected opportunities to bend down and pick up her treasures (we rarely notice exercise performed for pure pleasure).

Winged sycamore seeds, crimson, yellow and rust-coloured autumn leaves, sprays of honesty or lavender, rosemary or other herbs, swathes of long grasses, cow parsley and purple loosestrife are all there waiting for someone to notice them. As long as they are not protected, rare or poisonous (you must gen up of course) you could occasionally collect a few and arrange in water, dry, press, sketch and paint, make into herbal remedies, cosmetics or perfumes or turn into wall and table decorations. This can save you money on cut flowers, give you several new interests and hobbies and surprise friends who are more used to seeing the same types of flowers all the time and hear you complain that you are overworked and have nothing to do in your spare time!

If you live in a town or city, you could get in some bending by performing the neighbourly act of picking up sweet papers, cigarette ends or other litter. Whatever your choice, you now need your breakfast. For some healthy eating ideas, see below.

At 10.00 a.m. and throughout the day

Check your posture and drink a glass of water. If you've been sitting down for an hour or more, make sure that your feet are flat on the floor and your spine is comfortably extended and aligned. Imagine an invisible string running from the ceiling to the top of your head, gently easing your spine upwards to avoid undue stress on any joint or muscle. As often as you can, get up and walk about, take some deep breaths in front of a window or open the door and gently rotate your head and neck.

Elevenses

See the food and drink section later in the chapter and, if you haven't had a chance to venture outside yet, go now! If you are at home, get up and stretch, put the kettle on or pour yourself another glass of water. Take some deep breaths of fresh air standing outside or at an open window. Then, stretch up to the ceiling as though trying to reach it with your fingertips or simply follow the instructions for the Pilates shoulder drop and add the starfish for good measure (see page 56). Relax as you are doing these exercises – no one is timing you and they will only benefit you if you carry them out slowly and carefully enough to enjoy them.

If at work, don't forget that you are legally entitled to a break and it's up to you to make it work to your best advantage. Do the above exercises if you have the chance. If not, at least ensure that you get some fresh air into your lungs. You might even have enough time to perform a little step routine – especially if you can have the radio on. Try the simple one-step exercise – you could get several repetitions of this into around the same short spell it takes to read these suggestions! Clearly the suitability of these or any exercises during a working day depends on your environment and what you do in it. You obviously have more freedom of choice if you're a lighthouse keeper than a nurse in an intensive care unit! I am making these suggestions only to remind you of the many possibilities that exist for us, if we seek them out.

Lunchtime

This means food and drink, of course (see below), but equally important, a chance to counteract stress! Very few people deny feeling stressed at work, but if you really happen not to be, all I can say is 'Lucky you!' Chances are, though, that you'll feel so laid back and bored that you'll be falling asleep by the middle of the day. Whatever your perceived stress level, up and outside again you go. If it's really pelting with rain or blowing a gale, then you will either have to don some wet weather gear and brave the elements (this can actually be most refreshing) or nip off to the swimming baths to get in a few lengths (or widths) and wake yourself up.

The same applies if you are at home during the day, working for yourself, looking after children or whatever. If the latter, wrap them up and take them with you on your outside ventures. You can walk briskly if alone or with children of the right age or else become their age again for half an hour, playing It or Tag, beach (or park) cricket, kick the can or rounders, or simply chase the dog about (dogs need exercise too!). As noted before, what you do doesn't matter in the least, providing you enjoy it and it presents some challenge to your heart and lungs.

Afternoon break

I assume you have one of these whether you go out to work or not. Those 20 minutes mid-afternoon can be pleasurably spent ironing out postural creases (see Chapter 3), topping up your fluid levels, destressing, blowing away the cobwebs and using up a few calories. Did you think that they were just for lying back in your chair in your office or home and stuffing your face with cream cakes, chocolate bars or crisps? The effort and will power you may have to summon to say 'no' to these temptations will be amply rewarded by growing fitness, reduced aches and pains, fewer stress-related symptoms, such as depression, tension headaches and migraine, improved alertness and, very probably, sounder sleep, not to mention hugely increased self-esteem.

Don't forget, by mid-afternoon you are heading towards your evening reward (after a hard day's graft) of a chosen activity, recreation, eating and drinking and, above all for many of us, someone to natter to. You don't want to be too tired to enjoy these to the full.

Your evening

The best part of an evening (or weekend) for most people is the 'not having to do anything for anybody' aspect, having spent the day (or week) in the more or less willing service of others. You will serve your own purpose best, however, by including at least a few minutes of some sort of exercise before your evening meal, even if you have managed to fit some in during the day. This is particularly important if you have been desk- or chair-bound all day. It may be as simple as dancing around the room to a favourite tune while your meal cooks, walking the dog round the block, or getting in some yoga, Pilates or t'ai chi practice from a tape or book.

If you have had a stressful day, try to make sure that your evening activity is aerobic. Challenging heart, lungs and muscles really does enable you to let off steam and rid your system of all the pent-up irritations, frustrations and miseries the day has produced. This plan may also help if you tend to overeat or comfort eat as studies have shown that the endorphins and other hormones released by aerobic exercise help to suppress the appetite and make you feel happier.

Again, going for a swim on the way home may provide your perfect outlet. You could go for a brisk walk, to a jazz or belly-dancing class or horse riding, play half an hour of tennis with someone of the same standard or dig over a flower bed. Ripping off wallpaper (preferably in a room you had been intending to decorate!) provides a satisfaction all its own; and mowing the lawn, cutting hedges or tackling a local hill with just enough va va voom to make you slightly breathless, all have their devotees. Take the car to a suitable hill if it's more convenient!

No exercise – including the effortless variety – takes place in a vacuum. Its benefits will be much more apparent if you include it as part of an integrated and harmonious lifestyle (or as near this ideal as possible). All this means in practice is that enjoyable, energy-giving food and drink and adequate leisure time for socializing or pursuing other interests are every bit as important as exercise to your well-being. Indeed, they combine with it to promote the ultimate in physical, mental and emotional health.

Regular relaxation is particularly vital, and the way most of us start the winding-down process after a day's hard labour is by listening and chatting. Generally speaking, our families, partners, parents or friends can be relied on to listen interestedly as we relate the pleasures, sorrows, disappointments and joys that make up our days. They can also provide some much needed adult company if the day has been spent with small children. Listening to them in return can be rewarding, provide the chance for some laughter and help us to relax.

Bedtime

By the time you get into bed after a warm bath or shower, you should be feeling encouraged by all you have been able to fit into your day. However much or little you have achieved, it is another step further away from the couch potato's risk of early death and another one nearer to the health and vitality you deserve to enjoy. As you last exercised before your evening meal, the enhanced alertness this causes should have subsided by the time you go to bed, leaving you physically tired and ready for sleep.

If you still feel wide awake or suffer from insomnia anyway, here are some hints to help you drop off into a relaxing slumber:

- ensure that your bedroom is airy and cool without being chilly;
- make sure your bed is comfortable and noises are eliminated as far as possible;
- relax in the corpse asana (see page 48);
- read or listen to gentle music or a bedtime sound machine offering a range of tranquillizing sounds, from mountain streams, white noise or a fountain to a chorus of birds chirping and the sea;
- add a few drops of clary sage or chamomile essential oil to bathwater or to a carrier oil, such as almond, and use as a post-shower moisturizer;
- share a scented massage with your partner to double the pleasure;
- a milky drink last thing helps to induce sleep – the calcium soothes jangled nerves, while amino acids in the protein help to increase levels of endorphins and serotonin, which is the good mood brain chemical that combats anxiety and chronic pain, and induces sleep;
- make your bed a comforting refuge – change the bedlinen often and save up, if necessary, for the best goosedown pillows and duvet you can find for the ultimate experience in nocturnal cosseting;
- spritz your pillowcases with lavender (or rose) linen water or dab them with a couple of drops of the essential oils of these flowers, or of ylang ylang, chamomile or clary sage;
- relax all over with the light off, taking slow, deep, gentle breaths, gradually slowing the rate at which you exhale until it is taking twice as long as inhaling.

Food and drink

Our habits are highly personal. Giving up slothful habits on the exercise front will probably provide you with enough to cope with at first, without radically altering your diet too. It's true that some dietary adjustments early on may be advisable if one of your aims is weight loss. All the same, healthy changes in one direction very often lead, sooner or later, to similar changes in another. Feeling good about yourself for exercising regularly, for instance, may stem your emotional reliance on comfort foods, while aerobic exercise, as we have already seen, reduces the appetite and counteracts food cravings.

Nevertheless, I am including the following hints and tips on healthy eating and drinking to enhance the effects of your exercising and promote improved health and energy.

- Start each day with a glass of hot water and lemon juice for healthy skin and waste elimination. Add boiling water to a mug containing the juice of a lemon or lime plus a curl of its peel and leave to steep for ten minutes, covered. Sweeten with a teaspoon of honey or unrefined brown sugar if you find it is really too sharp for you (acclimatizing to the taste, though, reduces your sweet tooth for other foods).
- Drink at least eight medium tumblers of water every day. Tap or bottled water, mineral or spring, still or carbonated, it really doesn't matter, providing you get your 2 litres ($3\frac{1}{2}$ pints) plus in every day. Your need for water will increase in hot weather and when exercising. Ayurvedic health experts recommend room-temperature, still water as being best suited to the body's internal environment. Steer clear of large volumes of iced water immediately after aerobic exercise and when needing to boost your metabolism (that is, the rate at which your body burns fat). Warm or room-temperature fluids help to raise, or at least maintain, the metabolic rate.
- Eliminate alcohol altogether for a time if you frequently drink too much. Otherwise, reduce your intake to the recommended safe levels of 14 units a week for a woman or 21 for a man. A unit is 300 ml ($\frac{1}{2}$ pint) of 3 per cent alcohol-content beer or lager, a single measure of spirits or 100 ml ($3\frac{1}{2}$ fl oz) wine, which is a small glass).
- Choose your own level of caffeine intake. Too many 'don'ts' and 'cut downs' on the nutritional front make plaintive reading and are counterproductive – people then tend to do the opposite. Arguments against coffee, tea and cola drinks include links between caffeine and palpitations and *possibly* cancer of the breast, bowel and other areas, plus, of course, its diuretic action – that is, it increases urine production, which can be quite dehydrating, which is the opposite of the advice above to drink lots of water! Arguments in favour of caffeine drinks include their considerable 'comfort factor', increased alertness and the welcome loss of fluid for people who tend to retain it.

- Use fresh, dried and puréed fruit to add sweetness to dishes rather than 'pure, white and deadly' refined white sugar. Obviously you will consume some every day, but try to cut down on obvious sources, such as sweets and chocolate, jams, syrups and marmalade, biscuits and cakes, ice-cream, fizzy drinks, fruit juice and 'juice drinks', and manufactured desserts. Hidden sources can include tinned vegetables and other savoury products, fruit in 'light' syrup, cereals and cereal bars, tomato sauce, powdered coffee whitener, liquid coffee essence and fruit-juice flavoured mineral water. Bombarding your system with sugary snacks can lead to diabetes or, paradoxically, hypoglycaemia (low blood sugar) with shakiness, trembling, sweating, palpitations and faintness, especially during or after exercise, because the body gets used to these sudden hits of pure sugar, and this is in addition to the unwelcome effect of piling on the weight.
- Make sure you get your daily quota of five or more portions of fresh fruit and vegetables. Eat at least some of these raw, chewing them well to release antioxidant nutrients in their natural state. The fibre content in plant foods retards the release and absorption of fructose (fruit sugar), providing a safer and more prolonged source of available energy than sweets or chocolates, especially if eaten an hour or so before exercising.
- Grains (wheat, rye, oats, barley, corn, rice) in their unrefined forms, such as wholewheat pasta and bread, brown and wild rice, porridge, Westphalian rye bread, are an excellent source of energy as their starches are converted into natural sucrose. This, like fructose, is slowly released into the bloodstream following digestion, which is much better for the body than quickly released high levels of sugar. Pulses, seeds and nuts also provide energy in this way and all four of these food groups offer valuable sources of protein, plant oils, vitamins, minerals and trace elements.
- Meat-eaters are becoming increasingly aware these days of the need to cut down on saturated fat. Meat of almost every type – beef, lamb, pork, venison – makes for healthy eating, providing all visible fat and gristle are removed and healthy cooking methods are used. These include pot roasting, stir-frying, dry-frying, baking and steaming. The need for any additional fat can be met by substituting olive or groundnut oil (or similar) for lard and dripping.
- Alternative sources of first-class protein – that is, containing all the essential amino acid building blocks the body needs to obtain

from food – can be found in game, offal, poultry (remember to remove the fatty skin), eggs cooked without fat, cheese and fish. Oily fish, such as salmon, mackerel, tuna, trout and sardines, provide DEA and DHA, which are required by the brain cells for optimum functioning – hence the origin of the old wives' tale that 'fish makes you brainy'. Research has also shown that these two essential fatty acids relieve arthritic pain and significantly reduce the risk of suffering from Alzheimer's disease.

- Early morning stretches can be taken on an empty, or nearly empty, stomach. More vigorous exercise is best taken an hour or so prior to a main meal or an hour or so after a healthy snack of fruit, cereal, a wholemeal bread sandwich or other such small meals.
- Dairy products are not in themselves unhealthy. The body needs the calcium and other nutrients milk and its products provide, all of which are available in skimmed or semi-skimmed milk and low-fat yogurt and cheese. Healthier alternatives to butter include reduced-fat butter and vegetable oil mixtures flavoured with buttermilk and other butter-derived ingredients.

Some real-life experiences

There now follow some people's descriptions, in their own words, of the benefits they gained one, three or six months after making effortless stretch, resistance and aerobic exercises part of their more active lifestyles. Of course, no two people will experience precisely the same health effects even if they start with similar fitness levels and follow identical exercise programmes. These stages, therefore, are simply guidelines as to what you might reasonably expect. I hope they will spur you on towards greater health and vitality in your own life, whatever your sex, age or starting point – don't let anything put you off.

Jessie
Jessie is a teenager, aged 19.

'Six months ago, I hadn't exercised since playing with a skipping rope or ball around the age of nine. I liked watching the soaps on TV, playing games on my computer and sitting around chatting to my family or mates. I am not very tall and my weight went up out of proportion to my height – however often Mum asked me to walk our dog or go for a swim with her, I never would.

'Then Mum took me to the doctor's because I was always tired and exhausted and found myself puffing and panting when climbing hills or stairs. He said I was well, apart from being obese (hateful word – I was 4 stone (25 kg) overweight and my BMI was 32 – see pages 24–25). In the end I got sick of not being able to do anything – go dancing or for a proper walk with my friends – so Mum and I together took up effortless exercise.

'Not at all sure at first that I would stick with it, I started slowly with a five-minute brisk walk every other day. To my surprise I found I liked it, especially when a friend from school joined us and I did it with her instead of Mum. We progressed through 10- and 15-minute walks until we were walking for 20 to 30 minutes, three or four times a week. We went through a routine of simple stretches before and after our walks, and later joined a yoga group. We also incorporated some weights into our stretches – such as in squats and other gravity-defying stances – and used hand-held food tins several times a week.'

At one month 'I was already feeling fitter and less drowsy and sluggish – Mum said my friend Helen and I should congratulate ourselves: we had just completed the most challenging four weeks of our more active lifestyle. Like dieting and giving up smoking, it's only too easy to backslide after the novelty wears off. I felt good about myself, enjoyed the surprise and compliments of my friends and asked myself why – since exercise is so delightful – I had never taken it up before.

'Then the weather changed – or we felt *under* the weather; my life went through a brief bad patch when I failed my driving test and suddenly brisk walking lost its attraction. I longed for some comfort – old couch potato habits beckoned. I put my trainers back in the wardrobe (and my feet up on the coffee table in front of the television!), promising myself I would start again "when life picks up". Weasel words, you'll agree, but I fell for them right enough until I weighed myself and found that I had regained $\frac{3}{4}$ of the stone (5 kg) I had been so proud of losing. I was out on the streets in my trainers again next day.'

At three months 'I had shed 2 stone (13 kg); I was eating fairly sensibly and had cut out crisps, biscuits and chips between meals. Hills and stairs were far less challenging and Helen and I both had much more energy. Odd aches and pains I had noticed after prolonged sitting had disappeared. Our self-esteem and improving shapes boosted our social life and we both started to get noticed by boys.

'We met them generally socializing more because we took up volleyball to give us more aerobic workouts. We also went dancing and were never without partners – life was definitely looking up!'

At six months 'I had lost the third stone (6 kg) I was wanting to get rid of. Hills and stairs were no problem to us now – in fact, we barely noticed them. I felt bursting with energy, and even looked good in club gear when we went out at night. I looked and felt more toned all over and was starting to slink into evening gear as I had always dreamed of doing. I was much more flexible, as was Helen, because of our regular yoga. Even problem areas, such as my thighs and upper arms, though still a little plump, were starting to shape up due to squats and hand weights. I shed the final stone (6 kg) with the help of Weight Watchers and actually feel about ten years younger now than I did before I started effortless exercise.'

Susan
Susan, 34, is a busy mum.

'I believed for years that my busy lifestyle caring for three small children, my husband Rob, the home and a part-time job, provided all the exercise I needed. I shopped, cleaned, cooked, ferried the children to school and various activities and chased round after everyone at home. I was too exhausted to consider "extra" exercise as well! But I was aware of the many benefits exercise can bring and I did not feel I was getting them from the life I was leading. I was at least 20 pounds (9 kg) overweight, had yo-yo dieted and failed to lose weight and got puffed when I had to run for a bus. Our GP told me to exercise and cut down on fats because my blood pressure and cholesterol level were both raised. She said this might mean I could avoid taking drugs, which I was against anyway.

'I began with a brisk five-minute walk on alternate days, taking the children with me and linking up with another mum whenever possible. I also joined in the children's games more actively than before, taking a bat and ball or handball or football to the local park or playing with them in the garden. Five to ten minutes at a time were ample at first – running to hit or kick a ball, playing It or Tag and kick the can. This is a brilliant game like hide and seek, but more fun because those hiding have to sneak up on the person who is 'it' and kick a (preferably old and noisy) empty can as far as possible from a central clearing 'he' is guarding without being seen. If you are spotted, you become 'it' instead, so there is plenty of opportunity for movement.

My stretching exercise, at first, was a bit limited, but I soon started to enjoy the wonderful sensation of flexing and extending my body muscles, back, neck and limb joints.'

At one month 'I was already feeling a little fitter and life was beginning to be fun again. I patted myself on the back, I have to admit. It isn't easy to find time for regular exercise when you feel permanently bushed – especially with a family and job to attend to – but the more I play with the children, the more I find I can let myself go. The kids think it's a hoot – or "wicked" – and relish the extra contact. They are also benefiting from all the increased activity. I actually had more energy than before I started exercising and was sleeping more soundly too.

'Night and morning stretches soon started to show how stiff and painful my neck, shoulders and back get. I made more of a routine of them and sometimes got my husband to massage my sore bits after a relaxing bath. As I was sleeping better (and the delights of massage make themselves increasingly obvious), my sex drive – which had gone into a decline after our third baby – suddenly perked up again.'

At three months 'I was getting more active and energetic by the week! I could play, chase, jump about, skip for up to 10 to 15 minutes or longer without panting and sweating uncomfortably. All this additional fresh air and oxygen was improving my looks – my skin was clearer, complexion rosier, and previous tiredness bags under my eyes had long since disappeared. My sex drive continued to get better – Rob was, in fact, sufficiently impressed by the changes in me to want to join in the exercise. My only bugbear was a bad back – our GP put this down to lax muscles and poor posture during hours of driving and sitting at a desk. She gave me the all clear to try extra stretching, so I bought a yoga video and Rob and I learned this together. I often played masseuse, too, for Rob – using aromatherapy oils to heighten our shared pleasure.

'My surplus pounds dropped off, too, with the extra exertion – I easily regain weight, so I began walking briskly several times a week with my next-door neighbour.

At six months 'Wow! I was feeling and looking great! Podgy pounds had vanished and my self-esteem, confidence, get-up-and-go were back in abundance. Regular walking had slowed my pulse to a healthier rate and improved my breathing. I had long stopped picking at food and just enjoyed eating healthily. I never had smoked, but I used to drink a bit too much at times. I have dropped this habit, too (quite apart from other considerations, I am determined not to regain any surplus weight!).

'Rob and I also took up horse riding and badminton. We met new people and made new friends, and yoga was an established part of our daily routine – we felt we never, ever wanted to do without it! We also toned our muscles a couple of times a week with weight training at home, using any props to hand.'

Reggie
Reggie is now 53, but his life began again at 50.

'I was probably the most reluctant exerciser ever! Old habits die hard and the older they are, the harder they die! When I turned 50, I felt that all my useful years were behind me – my wife had just left me for a younger man, I was made redundant and I was full of aches and pains. The last thing I felt like was taking up exercise. However, my GP diagnosed depression and said my poor sleep was due to worry. He advised me to get more active. He is 60, plays golf, swims and is a third dan judo black belt, so he knows what he is talking about.

'I started effortless exercising, determined to give it a go, but not particularly hopeful as to the outcome. I was so conscious of being overweight and felt awkward, stiff and ancient. I watched our grandchildren running round – playing tennis, dancing, playing football and netball – and barely getting out of breath. Wouldn't I be making a fool of myself if I tried to do the same, after all these years?'

At one month 'I was already realizing that exercising for health is not competitive. Regular, gentle stretching, night and morning, relieved my aching back, shoulders, hips and knees. At first I became puffed simply from stretching, but my endurance improved when I included 10 to 15 minute walks in my daily routine. I started walking around the local park – I was a keen gardener and had never really taken much notice of the trees and flowers and shrubs on public display. They were something to look at and think about as I experimented with various routes to ring the changes.

'My muscles were still pretty flabby, but I did not worry about looks at this stage. What I did notice was that the daily routine plus fresh air (it was autumn) "got me going" – my depression lifted and I felt, having hit rock bottom, that the only way out was up. How right I was.'

At three months 'Yes!! By this stage I had included regular resistance routines into my daily stretches, and these were starting to define and tone my muscles. I was sleeping through the night and I had also lost a few pounds around the tummy region. And I have to say that an increased awareness of my posture not only put paid to backache and shoulder pain, it also made me look and feel taller and more slender. I was starting once again to take a pride in my appearance. Best of all, far from feeling foolish in front of the grandchildren, they became my champions! They get taught a lot of stuff about nutrition, exercise and how the body works at their school and the two older ones gave me dozens of ideas for healthy high-energy foods and how to cut down on cholesterol and saturated fats.

'They also organized long weekend rambles in the woods and fields between their homes and mine. "Taking Grandad walkies" became a family joke, until I knocked that one on the head by buying Ben, an abandoned fox terrier, from the local rescue centre. It then became all of us "taking Ben walkies", and I am pleased to say that he nearly ran *them* off their feet! Ben was, and is, the most wonderful companion, and I quickly became far less lonely. I have even started watercolour painting evening classes. Life is definitely looking up.'

At six months 'By this stage, exercising had become so much a part of my life that it seemed I had been doing it for ever. My backache had been reduced to the occasional twinge, my weight was right for my sex and height, and I felt fit as a flea. I occasionally got a bit depressed when I thought about the demise of my marriage (Annette and I had been together for 30 years), but it was nothing I couldn't cope with.

'Then a miracle happened. I met a very attractive lady a couple of years younger than me at the watercolour class. I learned that she, too, was divorced and, when she asked if I liked dogs, I told her how and why I had come to buy Ben. She admitted that she wanted to get back to exercising but had no one to exercise with. It was a small step to suggesting we walk our two hounds together (she lived down the road from me).

'Soon, we were walking round the park and in the country nearly every day and, after a couple of months, we decided to take up ballroom dancing again as we had both enjoyed this with our exes. Mary also started t'ai chi (yoga did not appeal to her) and persuaded me to join after she had done it for a term. We both liked it immensely and found t'ai chi excellent for posture, stretching, resistance, balance and combating stress. We moved in together a year ago and have never been happier. It's no exaggeration to say that all this came about because I acted on my doctor's advice and started exercising.'

Marjorie
Marjorie is 70 and has rediscovered yoga and the health benefits of exercising.

'I had no idea of the benefits exercise can give you when you are older, until I saw a TV programme about our need to stay active in advancing years. "Use it or lose it", the producer said, and this made plenty of sense – you only have to think how a stroke victim's muscles grow jelly-like and seem to wither once they are paralysed. This happened to my Wilf, and it was very sad as he had been a lumberjack in Canada in his youth and always stayed very fit – until the stroke.

'The figures mentioned in the programme shocked me. It seems that only 21 per cent of women and 32 per cent of men in the UK aged 55 to 64 take the recommended 30 minutes of exercise most days. Scottish people fare even less well, only 26 per cent of men and 21 per cent of women for this age group being sufficiently active. These figures fall even further beyond the age of 65 years, only 17 per cent of men and 12 per cent of women in the UK taking 30-minute exercise sessions on most days (in Scotland the figures are 14 per cent of men and only 8 per cent of women).

'Anyway, I heard about effortless exercise and decided to give it a go. I liked it because you can start ever so gradually – it would be a big mistake to pitchfork yourself into exhausting routines from the start. You'd probably put something out! I learned some yoga years ago and could remember most of the asanas – I really do not know why I gave it up! I did three or four of these for about 10 minutes on getting out of bed each day, to start with, and eventually built up to 20 minutes morning and night. I am lucky not to suffer from arthritis, although there are lots of poses you could do even with stiffish joints.'

At one month 'I was well into yoga again and enjoying every minute. I also started playing handball with my grandchildren. We enjoyed the time we spent together and I found my co-ordination, perhaps a bit shaky at first, had already improved (helped no doubt by the yoga). I did feel a sense of achievement! One tip I can pass on: make sure you wear the correct glasses if you use them or have your eyes checked if you are in doubt – balance is strongly affected by vision.

'Regular activity also boosted the circulation in my hands, legs and feet, which felt much warmer, and I stopped suffering from night cramps. I also slept better because I was no longer tossing and turning as a result of icy lower legs.'

At three months 'By now I was really in the swim of regular exercise – literally, because my sister and I took up aquarobics at the local swimming pool! They hold a class for the over fifties every week in term time. This made us both pant and puff a lot at first and we had difficulty keeping up, but so did a number of the other ladies – some far younger than we – so we just did the best we could. Eventually we could do all the instructor taught the class to do. She was most helpful and kind, and encouraged everyone of us in turn.

'We always went for a little swim afterwards – the resistance offered by the water helps to strengthen and tone your muscles and we both benefited. The other aerobic thing we did was a walk twice a week round the local golf course, setting our own pace, of course. I have to say, our complexions picked up no end – the fresh air and exercise brought roses to our cheeks and we both felt – and, I have to say also looked – about ten years younger.'

Further Reading

William Bird and Veronica Reynolds (2002) *Walking for Health and Happiness: The complete step-by-step guide to looking good and feeling your best*, Penguin Putnam.

Paul Brecher (2000) *T'ai Chi*, Thorsons First Direction series, Thorsons.

Garri Garripoli (1999) *Qigong: Essence of the healing dance*, Health Communications.

Cheryl Isaacson (2001) *Yoga*, Thorsons First Directions series, Thorsons.

Debbie Lawrence (1998) *The Complete Guide to Exercise in the Water*, A. & C. Black.

Lynne Robinson, Gordon Thomson and Helge Fisher (1999) *The Morning Energizer*, Pilates Through the Day series, Pan Books.

Useful Addresses

Age Concern England
Astral House
1268 London Road
London SW16 4ER
Tel: 0800 009966 (information line)
Website: www.ageconcern.org.uk
Ring for Staying Active publications and other exercise and health-related advice.

British Council for Chinese Martial Arts
c/o 110 Frensham Drive
Stockingford
Nuneaton
Warwickshire CV10 9QL
Tel: 0906 3021036
Website: www.bccma.org.uk

British Wheel of Yoga
25 Jermyn Street
Sleaford
Lincolnshire NG34 7RU
Tel: 01529 306851
Website: www.bwy.org.uk
E-mail: office@bwy.co.uk (for enquiries)

Pilates Institute
3rd Floor Wimborne House
151–155 New North Road
London N1 6TA
Tel: 020 7253 3177
Website: www.pilates-institute.co.uk

The Ramblers Association (main office)
2nd Floor Camelford House
87–90 Albert Embankment
London SE1 7TW
Tel: 020 7339 8500
Website: www.ramblers.org.uk

Zaida – belly dancing for older women, by Zaida and Phoebe K. Carter
Website: welcome.to/Zaida

Index